FRANCIE WOLGIN

ADVANCED SKILLS AND COMPETENCY ASSESSMENT FOR CAREGIVERS

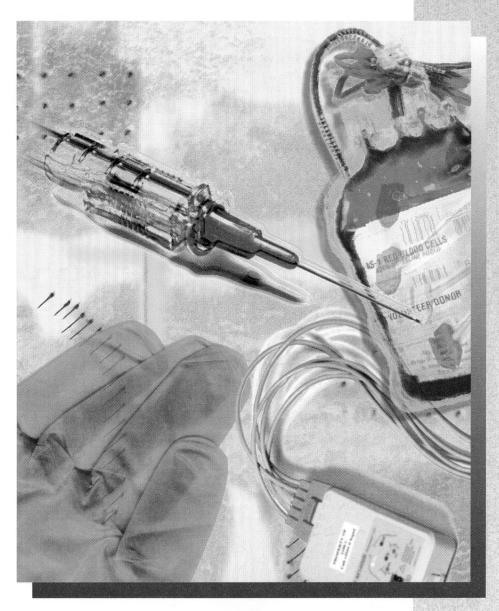

Foreword by
Sherry Makely

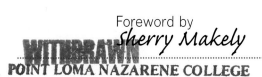

BRADY
PRENTICE HALL
Upper Saddle River NJ 07458

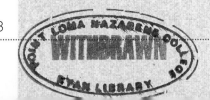

Library of Congress Cataloging-in-Publication Data

Wolgin, Francie.
   Advanced skills and competency assessment for
caregivers / Francie Wolgin
      p.   cm.
   Includes index.
   ISBN 0-8359-5167-7 (pb : alk. paper)
   1. Nursing—Examinations, questions, etc. 2. Care of the sick—
Examinations, questions, etc.   I. Title.
   [DNLM: 1. Caregivers—examination questions. 2. Nursing
Process—examination questions. WY 18.24 W861a 1997]
RT55.W63 1997
610.73′076—dc21
DNLM/DLC
for Library of Congress   97-34821
                                                                 CIP

Publisher: *Susan Katz*
Acquisitions Editor: *Barbara Krawiec*
Senior Managing Development Editor: *Marilyn Meserve*
Director of Manufacturing and Production: *Bruce Johnson*
Managing Production Editor: *Patrick Walsh*
Production Editor: *Susan Geraghty*
Production Liaison: *Cathy O'Connell*
Senior Production Manager: *Ilene Sanford*
Marketing Manager: *Judy Streger*
Marketing Coordinator: *Dori Steinhauff*
Editorial Assistant: *Stephanie Camangian*
Managing Photography Editor: *Michal Heron*
Photography: *Michal Heron*
Cover Design: *Joe Sengotta*
Cover Artwork: *Paul Gourhan*
Interior Design: *Amy Rosen*
Composition: *Carlisle Communications*
Printing and Binding: *Webcrafters*

© 1998 by Prentice-Hall, Inc.
A Simon & Schuster Company
Upper Saddle River, New Jersey 07458

Printed in the United States of America

10 9 8 7 6 5 4 3 2 1

ISBN 0-8359-5167-7

PRENTICE-HALL INTERNATIONAL (UK) LIMITED, *London*
PRENTICE-HALL OF AUSTRALIA PTY. LIMITED, *Sydney*
PRENTICE-HALL CANADA INC., *Toronto*
PRENTICE-HALL HISPANOAMERICANA, S.A., *Mexico*
PRENTICE-HALL OF INDIA PRIVATE LIMITED, *New Delhi*
PRENTICE-HALL OF JAPAN, INC., *Tokyo*
SIMON & SCHUSTER ASIA PTE. LTD., *Singapore*
EDITORA PRENTICE-HALL DO BRASIL, LTDA., *Rio de Janeiro*

NOTICE

The procedures described in this textbook are based on con-
sultation with nursing authorities. The author and publisher
have taken care to make certain that these procedures reflect
currently accepted clinical practice; however, they cannot be
considered absolute recommendations.

   The material in this textbook contains the most current
information available at the time of publication. However,
federal, state, and local guidelines concerning clinical practices, including without limitation, those governing infection
control and universal precautions, change rapidly. The
reader should note, therefore, that new regulations may
require changes in some procedures.

   It is the responsibility of the reader to familiarize himself
or herself with the policies and procedures set by federal,
state, and local agencies, as well as the institution or agency
where the reader is employed. The authors and the publish-
ers of this textbook, and the supplements written to accom-
pany it, disclaim any liability, loss, or risk resulting directly or
indirectly from the suggested procedures and theory, from
any undetected errors, or from the reader's misunderstanding
of the text. It is the reader's responsibility to stay informed of
any new changes or recommendations made by any federal,
state, and local agency as well as by his or her employing
health care institution or agency.

NOTE ON GENDER USAGE

The English language has historically given preference to the
male gender. Among many words, the pronouns, "he" and "his"
are commonly used to describe both genders. The male pronouns still predominate our speech; however, in this text "he"
and "she" have been used interchangeably when referring to the
Nursing Assistant and/or the patient. The repeated use of "he or
she" is not proper in long manuscript, and the use of "he or she"
is not correct in all cases. The authors have made great effort to
treat the two genders equally. Throughout the text, solely for the
purpose of brevity, male pronouns and female pronouns are
often used to describe both males and females. This is not
intended to offend any reader of the female or male gender.

*Dedicated in loving memory of Augusta Cohen, whose zest for
life and caring compassion inspired all who knew and loved her.*

$\mathcal{C}$ONTENTS

$\mathcal{C}$HAPTER 1

GROWTH, DEVELOPMENT, AND AGE-SPECIFIC CONSIDERATIONS   2

$\mathcal{C}$HAPTER 2

STANDARD PRECAUTIONS, ASEPSIS, AND STERILE TECHNIQUE   18

*C*HAPTER 3

*C*HAPTER 4

CHAPTER 5

CHAPTER 6

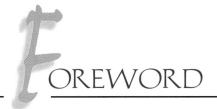

FOREWORD

As health care professionals and team members, each of us has an important role to play in delivering high-quality health care services for our patients. In this age of restructuring, downsizing, and cost cutting, getting the job done is no easy matter. We're increasingly challenged to do more with less, while maintaining and, it is hoped, improving the quality of care.

Everywhere we turn, things are changing. Health care providers who were once fierce competitors are now joining together to form large, integrated networks. Mergers, buyouts, and acquisitions leave employees wondering just who they work for. Managed care contracts, health maintenance organizations, and "gatekeepers" are becoming increasingly prevalent. Health care services are shifting to outpatient settings where primary care and health and wellness are gaining increased attention.

Probably nowhere is the impact of change felt more acutely than in hospitals. Fewer patients are admitted to hospitals today, and when they are, they stay fewer days. Hospitals have begun downsizing, closing patient care units, and reducing staffing levels. Many are undergoing restructuring, putting new care delivery models into place. This often results from using a "systems" perspective to determine how work processes must be changed based on the patient's point of view. Services like phlebotomy, ECG, pharmacy, and patient admitting and billing are often "decentralized" and relocated to patient care units.

The restructuring of hospitals is having a major impact on the health care workforce and the roles that workers play. All sorts of new job titles, job descriptions, and scopes of responsibility are emerging through work redesign. Never before have health care workers had such new, exciting opportunities for growth, and never before has lifelong learning been so crucial to their success.

The name of the game in health care today is flexibility. The more you know and are able to do, the better your chances of surviving and thriving. If you're reading this book because you've been given the opportunity to learn something new, go for it! Flexibility, versatility, and a willingness to acquire new skills now translate into enhanced value to your employer, along with higher levels of job security, marketability, and mobility.

A common element in work redesign is the use of cross-trained, or multiskilled, caregivers. Being multiskilled means that these caregivers can provide more than one function, often in more than one discipline. Just about everyone benefits from multiskilling. Multiskilled workers are flexible, versatile, and cost-effective—all the traits now in high demand among employers. In addition, multiskilled workers enjoy more variety and less routine, and they're better able to see the "big picture" of what's going on with each patient.

Employers who have more flexibility in the assignment of multiskilled workers may see productivity increase and labor costs decline. The number of "handoffs" needed to complete procedures decreases, so there are fewer steps in the process. Tests and treatments can be done faster, and decisions can be made more rapidly.

Multiskilling benefits patients, too, because they have fewer caregivers to interact with, and their care is better coordinated and more convenient. Because fewer caregivers are involved, there's less chance for duplication and error, and less time is spent waiting for specialists.

When workers are well trained and competent, multiskilling can have significant benefits. The benefits are evident not just in hospitals, but in health care facilities of all types, sizes, and locations. As you might imagine, the demand for multiskilled workers has been steadily growing over the past ten years, and now it's absolutely booming! In many facilities, willingness to be cross-trained is a condition of initial employment and a requirement of continued employment. Everyone—from patient caregivers, support staff, and business office workers—is affected by the demand for multiskilled workers.

Multiskilled workers are becoming especially prevalent on hospital patient care units. Many function as nurse "extenders," or partners who work on care teams with registered nurses. They often have generic, team-based titles, such as patient care technician, patient care assistant, clinical associate, unit technician, and care team member. Working under the direct supervision of RNs and other professional staff members, extenders take over some of the more basic and routine functions of patient care and testing. Although some RNs voice concerns about the growing use of these "unlicensed assistive personnel," many nurses who have worked with well-trained, competent extenders have come to rely on them. These caregivers are very valuable members of the health care team, but competency is vital! Extenders must be confident in their work, and so must everyone else who works with them. For this reason, thorough training and the assessment of competency are extremely important.

The key for health care employers today, especially in hospitals, is to adjust the "mix" of personnel to determine how many specialists, multiskilled workers, licensed personnel, and extenders are needed to get the job done (and done well) at a reasonable expense. The more workers know and are able to do, the better they fit into the new paradigm of health care. That's where you come in, and that's why this book is so valuable.

It's likely that you're reading this book for one of two reasons. Either you're a health care worker who is about to acquire some additional patient care skills, or you're an educator who needs an instructional tool to address some of today's training challenges. In either case, you've made a wise decision because *Advanced Skills and Competency Assessment for Caregivers* is an outstanding and innovative text geared to meet a variety of needs.

The author, Francie Wolgin, is nationally renowned for her expertise in training multiskilled workers and extenders for patient care units. With more than twenty-five years' experience as a registered nurse and professional educator, Francie knows what it takes to produce highly skilled, competent workers. She's the author of one of the nation's leading textbooks for nurse assistant training. Now, with *Advanced Skills and Competency Assessment for Caregivers,* she's gone one step farther to support advanced skills training among more experienced workers.

A unique characteristic of this text is its ability to meet the needs of a variety of learners. Unlike other books, it's not a "basic skills" text. Instead, it builds on whatever prior knowledge and skills learners bring with them. It facilitates the acquisition of new skills when they're needed, and it helps develop skill sets for a variety of different jobs and employment settings. It's precisely what health care calls for today.

This book serves the needs of a variety of learners, from nurse assistants and multiskilled patient care technicians to allied health professionals and experienced nurses who wish to extend their expertise. It's also a valuable learning tool for RN and LPN/LVN educational programs, for staff development educators orienting new program graduates once on the job, and for continuing education and cross-training caregivers. It also serves as an excellent reference book for follow-up after training.

Material is presented in a user-friendly fashion, but it goes into greater detail for complex skills than do the more basic texts. Acknowledging that many people learn best through visual images, the text includes more than two hundred colored drawings and photographs to enhance readability and learner comprehension. Detailed, step-by-step instructions walk learners through each procedure with objectives, key terms, supplies and equipment lists, and pertinent information all provided. One of its most valuable features is its emphasis on age-specific considerations for skills and procedures.

If you're an educator, one of your favorite components of this text is likely to be its competency assessment tools. As we all know, competency assessment and documentation of skills are becoming increasingly important, especially because of variations in the educational backgrounds, experience, and skill sets of workers.

Let's face it—time is limited, so why reinvent the wheel? Instead of each health care facility designing its own competency standards and assessment tools, this text provides a great place to start. Using the computer disk available for your convenience, you can easily customize the assessments to meet your specific institution's needs. With some fine-tuning, staff development specialists, preceptors, and instructors will be ready to check off skills and validate competencies for the variety of different staff members who perform each procedure. These tools are also useful in assessing the skills of program graduates, new employees, and workers who need annual competency documentation.

What are others saying about this book?

"It's user-friendly, and the visuals really help with learning."

"It covers topics that haven't always been well covered in the past."

"This is exactly what our staff development department needs!"

"I like the stand-alone chapters that can be mixed and matched as needed."

"I don't always have the depth of knowledge in each procedure that I wish I had, so as an educator, this makes my job a lot easier."

To learners preparing to read this book, congratulations on your opportunity to acquire some new and advanced skills. The more you know, the better. This text will be a big help to you. To educators adopting this text for training and assessment, you're making a wise decision. This book can save you lots of time and ensure success for your learners.

Thanks to Francie Wolgin, her clinical colleagues, and Brady/Prentice Hall for creating this book for us.

Sherry Makely
PH.D, RT-R, DIRECTOR

ADD-A-COMP® Program and Worker Retraining
Clarian Health Partners, Inc./Methodist Hospital
INDIANAPOLIS, INDIANA

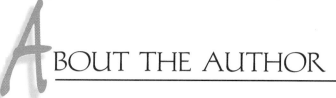 ABOUT THE AUTHOR

Francie Wolgin, MSN, RN, CNA

Francie Wolgin, MSN, RN, CNA, is director, Operations Support and Practice Development, St. Joseph Mercy Hospital, Ann Arbor, Michigan, and president, National Nursing Staff Development Organization. Her St. Joseph Mercy department is responsible for the training and development of all patient care associates including orientation and ongoing competency assessment of nurses and the patient care assistant and patient care technician training programs. Ms. Wolgin also serves as adjunct faculty at the University of Michigan School of Nursing.

Ms. Wolgin's previous positions include director of Nursing Practice Development and clinical associate, School of Nursing, Duke University Medical Center, and several management, staff development, and administrative positions at the University of Cincinnati Hospital and College of Nursing and Health faculty appointment. Ms. Wolgin serves on the *Journal of Nursing Staff Development* editorial board and is the department editor for *Perspectives on Research*. She also serves on the national advisory board for the Cross County University. She wrote *Being a Nursing Assistant,* 7th ed., as well as many articles and contributes to books on staff development, competency, and training advanced nursing assistants. Considerable experience as a direct caregiver in a variety of positions and areas provides both perspective and first-hand knowledge of the challenges and opportunities available throughout the health care continuum.

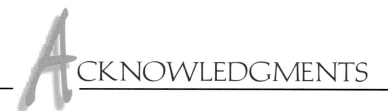ACKNOWLEDGMENTS

For their contributions to individual chapters, I gratefully thank the following:

Cherie Biscupski, BSN, RN, CCRN, education coordinator, Cardiology and Thoracic Surgery, St. Joseph Mercy Hospital, Ann Arbor, Michigan. Basic ECG, 12 Lead, and ACLS instructor. (Chapter 6)

Lisa Friedman, MS, RN, education specialist, St. Joseph Mercy Hospital, Ann Arbor, Michigan. Chapter contributor and coauthor of *Being a Nursing Assistant,* 7th ed., Instructor Guide; previous nursing instructor, Madonna University, Livonia, Michigan; and coordinator patient care assistant and PCT program, Ann Arbor, Michigan. (Chapters 1, 3, 4, 6)

Amy Larson, MS, RN, CNRN, CS education coordinator, St. Joseph Mercy Hospital, Ann Arbor, Michigan. Chapter contributor for *Being a Nursing Assistant,* 7th ed. Coordinates and teaches PCA and PCT training and RN orientation. Participated in the NIH Neuroscience Nurse Internship Program. (Chapter 2)

Mary Morocknick, BA, RN, nurse manager, IV chemotherapy team and rehabilitation unit, Duke University Medical Center. Chapter contributor for *Being a Nursing Assistant,* 7th ed. (Chapter 5)

Marcia Sherman, RN, education coordinator, MICU and Medicine, St. Joseph Mercy Hospital, Ann Arbor, Michigan. Basic ECG and BLS instructor. (Chapter 6)

Jan Treston-Aurand, MS, RN, CIC infection control practitioner, St. Joseph Mercy Hospital, Ann Arbor, Michigan. Chapter contributor for *Being a Nursing Assistant,* 7th ed. (Chapter 2)

Brady/Prentice Hall

Susan Katz, publisher, for her initiative, openness to a creative approach to competency assessment, and support throughout the project.

Marilyn Meserve, managing development editor, for providing hands-on commitment, zealous energy, and coordination.

Stephanie Camangian, editorial assistant, for providing assistance and editorial support.

Patrick Walsh, managing production editor, and the in-house production team, including **Cathy O'Connell,** who provided production expertise and coordinated those aspects associated with the book's production.

Judy Streger, marketing manager, for her ongoing support.

Judy Stamm, Brady sales manager, and each member of the Brady sales team, for their support, suggestions, and sales promotion.

Susan Geraghty, project editor, for her editing skill, understanding of the project's vision, and support related to the technical production details.

Judith Mara Riotto, copyeditor, for her attention to detail and enhancing suggestions.

Michal Heron, managing photography editor, dedicated to capturing each desired photograph and choosing the best presentation. It was a pleasure hosting the photography shoot and being exposed to the nuances of photography.

St. Joseph Mercy Hospital, Ann Arbor, MI

Special thanks to Garry Faja, CEO, and Harriette Ehnis, interim executive management patient care director, for their support throughout the project and giving permission to reprint or adapt within this book and its supplements materials and forms from St. Joseph Mercy Hospital. I would also like to acknowledge Rosemary Kucharek, phlebotomy section leader, Clinical Laboratory, for her assistance and information related to blood specimen collection competency assessment, and Valerie Moore, RN, Jean Hirt, BSN, RN, and Judy Meyers, MS, RN, for their contributions to the adult and geriatric age-specific competencies. Special thanks to everyone at St. Joseph Mercy Hospital who facilitated and participated in the photo shoot, especially Nan Curtis and Lisa Marshall, who assisted with preparing the photography and art specs. The sterile procedure checklist was contributed by Michelle Diepenhorst, BSN, RN.

Technical Advisors

Thanks to the following people for providing technical support during the photo shoots.

Curtis Donald
Patient care technician

Lisa Friedman, MS, RN
Education specialist

Keith Jackson
Patient care technician

Amy Larson, MS, RN, CNRN
Education coordinator

JoLynn Pulliam, MS, RN, CPHQ
Education specialist

Marcia Sherman, RN
Education coordinator

Reviewers

Sonja Anderson, RN, C
Inservice education director
Angel Medical Center
Franklin, NC

Terry Ainsworth, MS, RN
Duke University Medical Center
Durham, NC

Judy Baker
Director of education, Education Department
Columbia Valley Regional Medical Center
Brownsville, Texas

Marian Beck Clore, RN
Director of staff development
Department of Staff Development
Doctors Hospital of Jackson
Jackson, MI

Shari Gould, RN
Education coordinator
Yoakum Community Hospital
Yoakum, TX

Tammy Jo Hill, RN, CEN, CCRN, EMT
Staff nurse and staff educator
Emergency Department
Russell County Hospital
Russell Springs, KY

Catherine E. Knight, RN
Clinical educator
Educational Services Department
Mercy Center for Health Care
Aurora, IL

Rosemary Kucharek
Phlebotomy section leader
Clinical Laboratory
St. Joseph Mercy Hospital
Ann Arbor, MI

Russell Olmstead, MPH, CIC
Department of Infection Control Services
St. Joseph Mercy Hospital
Ann Arbor, MI

Penney Parker, RN
Director of Education
Natchez Community Hospital
Natchez, MS

Edwina M. Rader, RN
Manager
Education, Training, and Research
Passaic Beth Israel Hospital
Passaic, NJ

Sandy Taylor, RN, BSN, CCRN
Director of Critical Care and Education
Critical Care and Education Department
Norton Community Hospital
Norton, VA

Linda A. Williams
Director, Education and Organizational Development
Columbia Presbyterian Hospital
Oklahoma City, OK

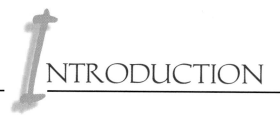

INTRODUCTION

Welcome to *Advanced Skills and Competency Assessment for Caregivers*. This book responds to identified needs and challenges in health care today. Educators are expected to develop programs to cross-train staff and/or provide orientation for new employees to competently perform a variety of skills. Variations in practice patterns occur from state to state because there are no consistent national standards. Therefore, educators adhere to the standards and expectations applicable to their practice setting. A basic premise of this book is that although there are variations in how caregivers may be trained to provide a given skill, there should be consistency in the assessment of their competency to perform each skill. Educators and caregivers will find that there are frequent changes or advances in health care as a result of research studies, clinical outcome measurements, insights, equipment changes, or new technology. Your instructor or preceptor will have the most current knowledge, and will adapt the competency validation to reflect the practice in your practice setting, agency, or state.

This book is designed to provide educators, preceptors, and caregivers a framework for competency assessment related to skill acquisition. There are six individual chapters that are designed to stand alone for the purpose of cross-training a variety of health care professionals, or they can serve as a foundation for many of the required skills expected of multifunctional workers.

Each individual skill includes its purpose, supplies needed, key terms, key information, and appropriate age-specific implications. The key concept is stressed in places where it is helpful to reinforce retention. The procedure for each skill is frequently complemented by photographs or drawings. Most important, there are competency validation checklists. The caregiver will be able to demonstrate the skill and the preceptor will be able to use the checklists to verify this in writing. The competency validation can become part of an individual record or serve as evidence that a particular competency has been demonstrated. Instructors, preceptors, or staff development educators can use a specially created disk to modify the competencies as necessary for their practice setting.

OVERVIEW

Chapters 3 through 6 in this book are designed to offer a foundation of advanced skills based on a knowledge of age-specific considerations and developmental tasks for infants through older adults (found in Chapter 1) and Standard Precautions and aseptic and sterile techniques (found in Chapter 2). Competency related to the procedures can be assessed and validated on the checklists. Procedures tend to have a series of steps that occur in a particular order. There is limited variation in how one employs Standard Precautions or protective equipment, for example. Guidelines, however, may be seen as more flexible recommendations, and as such may be carried out with more caregiver variation. There may be several ways to correctly perform an activity when the outcome is the same.

Chapters 3 through 6 include a variety of advanced patient care skills. Skills imply the effective application of knowledge along with ready execution, coordination, or manual dexterity. Each advanced skill is outlined and followed by an individual competency validation. Some skills are more easily described than others. For those skills in which more in-depth information has been deemed necessary, the information is presented before the skill is described. Examples include vein selection, ECG monitoring, and arrhythmia recognition. Many caregivers have not had exposure to this material and will require time to study and review the material. This book is a resource for them to study and review the skill steps.

C O N T E N T S

All chapters and main section headings as well as procedures, guidelines, and skills are listed in the contents.

Introduction

A paragraph at the beginning of each chapter highlights the content and skills to be included in each chapter.

Purpose

The reason why you want to perform a skill is located at the beginning of each skill. Frequently patients ask caregivers what they are doing or why it is necessary. Putting this information or skill description first provides a framework for the skill. If you do not understand what you are trying to accomplish, it is difficult to describe it to someone else.

Key Terms

Listed in the beginning of each chapter or following the objectives in each skill are key terms that are used in the chapter or skill description. Learning or reviewing the meaning of these terms before reading the chapter will greatly increase your understanding of the content and improve your ability to remember what you learn. Key terms are printed in bold followed by their definition.

Objectives

Each skill begins with a list of objectives that describe what the caregiver will be able to do in measurable, reachable goals: procedures or tasks to be performed, guidelines or techniques to be followed, or information to be reported or documented.

Supplies/Equipment

A list of the supplies or equipment needed to perform a skill are included.

Pertinent Points

Information, suggestions, or important patient considerations are listed in each skill.

Age-Specific Considerations

Most skills have important age-specific considerations that need to be taken into account when performing the skill. When appropriate these are included in this section.

Key Concepts

Key concepts are the most vital pieces of information you want to keep in mind as you perform a given skill. Frequently patient safety, well-being, and/or successful skill completion are dependent on the key concept.

Steps

Each step is listed in order along with photographs or drawings or a visual description of a particular aspect of a skill to assist in comprehension.

Competency Validation

Each skill offers a list to validate skill competence or progress toward competence. When acquiring new complex skills, sometimes caregivers do not find enough experiences available to attain competence.

Competence can be validated, or the form can be used to document progress. Competency validation has become increasingly important in health care settings or agencies. Acquiring advanced skills or cross-training benefits caregivers who are flexible and open to learning. There is a demand for these talents and skills in a variety of workplace settings. It is my hope that this book will be valuable to educators, preceptors, and caregivers who need to acquire, achieve, and document advanced skill competency. Patients and their families trust and rely on us to provide a standard of quality in our care delivery. Job titles of individual caregivers will vary, but the skill, competence, performance technique, and caring compassion should be the same. The need to document orientation and competency demonstration for external accreditation bodies and reviewers has gained emphasis in practice. However, the most important reason to validate competency is that each individual deserves and should expect no less than competent caregivers. A great deal of effort and collaboration have gone into developing this book to support and assist educators and managers who have more challenges than time.

Francie Wolgin

ADVANCED SKILLS AND COMPETENCY ASSESSMENT FOR CAREGIVERS

Chapter 1

Growth, Development, and Age-Specific Considerations

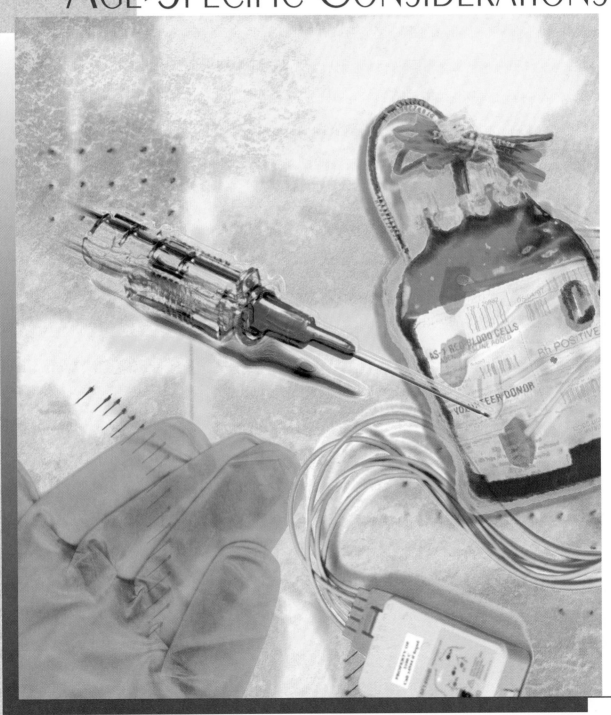

*O*ne of the most basic philosophies of health care is the recognition of each patient as an individual. Individual patients experience and express illness, injury, symptoms, and conditions in different ways in response to many factors. One of these factors is the age of the patient. This chapter describes normal growth and development skills over the course of the human life span. The goal is to allow the caregiver to place a patient's response to illness or injury within a range of what might be considered normal for the patient's age. Growth and development skills have a direct effect on patients' adjustment to illness or injury and on their ability to perform the tasks of their developmental age.

This discussion of growth and development also considers the issue of caregiver competence. *Competence* refers to the caregiver's ability to perform at an expected level to best meet the needs of the patient. In relation to age, caregivers are considered to be competent when they can adjust their caregiving behavior and communication style to best suit the particular age needs of the patient. This flexibility on the part of the caregiver helps the patient adjust to illness or injury and demonstrates respect and care for the patient.

This chapter prepares caregivers to do the following:

1. Identify normal growth and developmental trends in infants, toddlers, preschoolers, school-age children, and adolescents.

2. Identify skills acquired in the various developmental stages over the course of the human life span.

3. Describe the developmental tasks of the various age groups.

4. Recognize age-related factors that affect and influence patient care.

Chronological Age Actual age in years and months.

Cognitive Related to the mental processes by which knowledge is acquired.

Development The motor, language, cognitive, and social skill changes that occur over the course of the human life span.

Fine Motor Related to the movement of small muscles, such as those in the fingers and hands.

Gross Motor Related to the movement of large muscles, such as those used in walking or hitting a ball.

Growth The physical changes that take place over the course of the human life span as a person increases in size, as determined by weight, height, and other measures.

Growth and Development

Growth

Physical growth can be described as the total of many dynamic changes that occur as an organism increases in size, as measured by weight, volume, or linear dimension. In humans, this process begins at conception, and continues throughout life. These physical changes are measured in inches and pounds. In humans, however, growth is not limited to the physical dimension, but also includes the intellectual, social, and emotional growth processes as well. These processes occur from infancy to death.

Development refers to the acquisition and refinement of skills that allow the individual to adapt to the environment. They begin at a simple level and are refined at more complex levels all through the life span. Examples of these skills include motor abilities (crawling, walking, running), language skills, cognitive skills, and social skills.

Growth and development usually occur over predictable stages. Although growth and development occur at the same time, they occur at different rates for different individuals. Certain tasks must be mastered before progressing to the next developmental level. These tasks are generally grouped according to age as a reflection of the interaction between growth and development.

Chronological Age

Chronological age is the actual age of an individual measured in years and months. Patterns of growth for a given age are predictable within a range. For humans, growth begins at the time of conception. The first cell multiplies and divides, leading to the formation of all the tissues, organs, and structures of the body. This period, the prenatal period, takes 40 weeks. This is a time of extremely rapid growth. Once the infant is born, growth continues at a rapid pace for the first year of life. The following paragraphs describe typical patterns of human growth.

Infants: birth to 1 year After 40 weeks in the womb, infants are delivered into the world. Babies gain on average 1 to 1½ pounds a month, doubling their weight in the first six months. Growth continues at a rapid rate, with the average infant's weight tripling by the end of the first year. Babies also grow in length, and by their first birthday will be 50 percent longer than at birth.

An important measure of the growth of infants is the circumference of the head. This measurement of the distance around the baby's head is taken at the forehead. It indicates how fast the baby's skull, and therefore the brain, is growing. A circumference that is too small or too large may indicate serious medical problems.

What is most important about the growth of infants is that it be in proportion. Infants are monitored closely to see if their height, length, and head circumference are all increasing at the same rate, indicating normal growth.

Toddlers: 1 to 2 years The growth of toddlers is somewhat slower than that of infants. The average toddler gains 4 to 6 pounds a year, and the growth in height slows to about 3 inches per year. The growth in height is seen more in the elongation of the legs than in the trunk. By the age of two years, toddlers are approximately half of their adult height. During the toddler years, the measurement of head circumference is usually not obtained unless a problem was noted earlier.

Preschoolers: 2 to 5 years The growth of preschoolers is quite similar to that of toddlers. The average preschooler continues to gain 4 to 6 pounds a year and grows about 3 inches per year. Differences can be noted in how the body grows. Most of the growth in length appears to be in the elongation of the trunk instead of the legs, giving the preschooler the appearance of being taller and thinner than the toddler.

School-age children: 5 to 12 years The growth of the school-age child continues on a scale similar to that of the toddler and preschooler. Weight increases by 4 to 6 pounds per year, and height increases at a slightly slower rate of about 2 inches per year. Girls and boys follow similar patterns of growth from birth until the end of this period. As girls near their teenage years, they often grow taller and weigh more than boys of the same age.

Adolescence: 12 to 18 years It is during the teenage years that humans experience their second rapid growth period. Boys and girls grow almost as rapidly as they did as infants. This growth spurt generally occurs about two years earlier for girls than for boys. The period of adolescence spans a wide range from 12 to 18, reflecting the individuality for which growth occurs in each person. Both girls and boys experience physical and sex-specific changes (reproductive organs become functional for both sexes) during adolescence. Girls grow from 4 to 12 inches and gain from 15 to 55 pounds during this time. Boys grow 2 to 8 inches per year and gain 15 to 65 pounds during this time.

Young, middle, and older adults: 18 to 65+ years By the age of 18, most physical growth is complete, and wisdom teeth may erupt. After the age of 18, most new growth occurs in response to repairing the body after injury. As the individual gains in years, the signs of aging can be noted. In the absence of illness, aging is a fairly benign process. The biological changes of aging result in a diminishing of the senses: decreased sensitivity to smell, taste, sight, sound, and touch. A diminished reaction time is sometimes noted but does not correlate to the accuracy of the performance of a given task. Changes are gradual and occur at different rates for different individuals. Illness is not a normal part of aging. One of the goals of science continues to be to learn more about the human body and how it ages. This will allow for healthier individuals throughout the life span.

Development

Development refers to a wide range of motor, language, cognitive, and social skill changes and tasks that the individual masters and refines over the course of a lifetime. These skills are necessary and characteristic of humans. There are several different kinds of development. Cognitive development refers to the mental process through which humans gain knowledge. Social development refers to the process through which they gain skills to interact with one another. Language skills are the development and mastery of verbal and written communication processes. Fine-motor development involves the mastery of the movement of the small muscles in the hands and fingers. Gross-motor skills involve the mastery of the large muscles that control walking, running, throwing a ball, and so on. The mastery of all of these types of development is incremental and predictable for the various age groups.

Humans build on the skills they learn as infants and refine them as they grow. Infants are born possessing mastery of few developmental skills. Their parents interpret their needs and signals in order to care for them and protect them. Infants vocalize and imitate sounds. Toddlers can say "mama" and "dada," while preschoolers and school-age children are able to express a whole array of words and sentences.

Although growth is linked to age, it does not always follow an exact pattern. For example, most infants will be walking by their first birthday, but the range for the development of this skill is from 9 to 16 months. Therefore, age and developmental tasks for infants and toddlers may overlap. Developmental tasks are considered to be mastered when the individual can perform them most of the time.

Working with geriatric patients requires knowledge of a different set of skills. The caregiver must take into consideration physical limitations, unique psychosocial needs, and age-related illnesses.

Human development follows predictable patterns throughout the life span. Table 1.1 provides a brief description of these activities.

TABLE 1.1 DEVELOPMENTAL TASKS AND CHRONOLOGICAL AGE

Skill Area	Infant: Birth–1 Year	Toddler: 1–2 Years	Preschool: 2–5 Years	School-Age Child: 5–12 Years
Cognitive	Learns about new things by feeling and working with objects encountered in immediate environment and by placing or trying to place those objects in mouth	Expands knowledge of things by learning words associated with objects in environment	Comprehends tired, hungry, and other bodily experiences Recognizes colors	Learns relationship of objects to other objects and to self Learns relationship between objects and feelings
Social	Attaches to primary caregiver(s) Begins to recognize faces and smile; at about 6 months begins to recognize primary caregiver(s) and expresses fear of strangers Plays simple interactive games like peekaboo and patty-cake	Learns self and primary caregiver(s) are different or separate from each other Undresses self Imitates and performs tasks seen in environment Expresses needs or indicates wants without crying	Begins to separate easily from caregiver(s) Dresses with supervision Washes and dries hands Plays interactive games like tag	Acts independently, but is emotionally close to caregiver Performs work and gets rewarded for it Dresses without supervision Forms same-sex play groups and clubs
Language	Vocalizes, squeals, and imitates sounds Says "dada" and "mama"	Says three words other than *dada* and *mama* Follows simple instructions	Names one picture Follows directions Combines words to make simple sentences of two or three words; uses plurals Gives first and last names	Defines words Knows and describes what things are made of
Gross Motor	Lifts head first, then chest Rolls over, pulls to sit, crawls, and stands alone	Walks well, kicks, stoops, and jumps in place Throws balls	Runs well, hops, pedals tricycle Balances on one foot	Skips, balances on one foot for 10 seconds Overestimates physical abilities
Fine Motor	Reaches for objects and rakes up small items Grasps rattle Feeds self crackers	Unbuttons clothes Builds tower of 4 cubes Scribbles Uses spoon Picks up very small objects	Buttons clothes Builds tower of 8 cubes Copies simple figures or letters, for example *o* Begins to use scissors	Draws person with 6 parts Copies detailed figures and objects

Adolescent: 12–18 Years	Young Adult: 18–40 Years	Middle Adult: 40–65 years	Older Adult: 65+ Years
Understands abstract concepts like illness and death	Fully developed Continues to develop knowledge base related to school or job	Fully developed	Fully developed
Experiences turmoil with rapidly changing moods and behavior Demonstrates interest in peer group almost exclusively Distances from parents emotionally Expresses concern with body image Experiences falling in and out of love	Establishes independence from parents Forms an individual lifestyle Adjusts to companions Selects a career Copes with career, social, and economic constraints Chooses a mate Learns to live cooperatively with mate Becomes a parent	Builds socioeconomic status Assists younger and older people to cope Is fulfilled by work or family or by giving or caring for others Copes with physical changes of aging Relates to grown children and empty nest Deals with aging parents Copes with the death of parents	Develops mutually supportive relationships with grown children Adjusts to retirement Adjusts to loss of friends and relatives Copes with loss of spouse Forms new friends Adjusts to new role in family Copes with dying
Uses increased vocabulary Understands more abstract concepts like grief	Fully developed	Fully developed	Fully developed
May appear awkward while learning to deal with rapid increases in size due to growth spurts	Fully developed	Begins to experience physical changes of aging, such as decreased energy and endurance	Experiences more significant physical changes associated with aging
Fully developed	Fully developed	Fully developed	Begins to experience physical changes associated with aging

S E C T I O N   T W O
Age-Specific Considerations

Age-Related Care

To provide age-related, or age-specific, care to patients, it is vital that the caregiver understand and be able to adapt communication techniques and physical interventions to best meet the needs of each patient. Each individual responds to illness and injury in a unique way, based in part on the patient's age and the developmental skills he or she has mastered. The caregiver must develop different skills for assessing, treating, and teaching about illness and injury for the various age groups, or the outcome for the patient will not be the best. Figure 1.1 shows the communication, comfort, and safety considerations for the various age groups. Meeting patients' age-related needs shows them that they are respected and increases their trust in their caregiver.

Competence of care requires that the caregiver be able to assess the special needs and behaviors of each patient. It also requires that the caregiver have the necessary skills to provide care and have the ability to apply the principles of growth and development appropriately. For example, patients in neonatal or pediatric units do not have the skills and abilities to understand the treatment being given to them or the skills and abilities to adequately communicate their reactions and responses to treatment. These young patients often express themselves through nonverbal methods. Caregivers who work with these patients must be able to assess and care for them by understanding their unique needs and interpreting their nonverbal communications (Table 1.2).

Caring for adolescent patients often requires a different set of skills. Caregivers have learned that an authoritarian approach is not likely to be successful. This reflects adolescents' growing need to assert their independence and decision-making skills.

Working with geriatric patients requires knowledge of a different set of skills. The caregiver must take into consideration the physical limitations, unique psychosocial needs, and age-related illnesses of older adults. As individuals age, many physical changes occur that make independent functioning increasingly difficult. The body's central nervous system slows down, which could create problems in detecting heat, pain, and cold and could cause slower reflexes. Thought processes might be slow, and memory might become poor. All senses (hearing, sight, touch, taste, and smell) might be less sharp than they once were. Muscle tone might be poor due to lack of exercise and muscle atrophy. A disturbed sense of balance might make older adults unsteady on their feet or might cause a change in walking patterns. The bones tend to become brittle and break easily. Quick changes in position can cause blood pressure to drop, leaving the older patient feeling faint or dizzy. Posture might become stooped. Circulation becomes less efficient, and bodily processes slow down. The skin loses elasticity and some fat. The elderly might chill more easily due to the loss of body fat and decreased circulation.

One important point is that each individual is unique. A physician or nurse routinely performs patient assessments to determine what physical or psychological changes have occurred and whether certain aspects of care require modification.

Illness

The development of illness can have a profound effect on patients' ability to use the developmental skills they are learning or have already mastered. Illness often causes patients to function at a developmental stage they had already surpassed. For example, a hospitalized toddler might suddenly demand a bottle, or a preschooler who is toilet trained might suddenly regress and begin wetting the bed. The caregiver's role in such cases is to reassure the parents that this behavior is a common reaction to illness and will usually resolve itself once the illness has passed. Children who are hurting or anxious often revert back to behaviors that made them feel comfortable and safe at an earlier age. The caregiver can support the parents and the child by addressing their fears and anxieties.

Look on page 17 for an example of competencies caregivers should demonstrate when caring for adolescents and adults of all ages. In the elderly, illness can have a devastating effect on their ability to cope with age-appropriate developmental tasks. The fear of dependence and anxiety over the possible loss of friends, family, or home can have a profound effect on the ability of older patients to learn new skills for caring for themselves. The caregiver should allow geriatric patients to express these concerns and must support them in learning new skills and new behavior to promote healthier living and to assist them in maintaining their independence and as active a life as possible.

Injury

Injury can also have a profound effect on patients' ability to use the developmental skills associated with their chronological age. For example, a head injury can cause an active teenager to revert to the developmental level of a toddler, forcing the patient to relearn many of the skills of that age: talking, walking, dressing, bathing, and so on. Another example of a debilitating injury is a stroke, which might require an adult to relearn how to walk and talk. These types of injuries are extremely frustrating for patients. It might be difficult for them to use the calm, logical thinking processes they had previously used to solve a problem. Instead, they might lash out and throw something across the room in frustration with the slow progress their body is making. Review Table 1.2, which charts the appropriate caregiver behaviors associated with the different age groups. These behaviors will help patients understand and cope with their illness or injury in age-appropriate ways.

S U M M A R Y

All humans follow a similar path of growth and development, which progresses in stages. Each individual, however, moves through these stages in his or her own way. By understanding and knowing how humans grow and develop, caregivers can modify their care to best meet the health care needs of their patients.

	Communication	Comfort	Safety
NEONATAL **0 - 6 Months**	• Introduce yourself to caregiver. • Explain procedures to caregiver.	• Keep patient warm and dry. • Allow for usual feeding schedule. • Do not keep patient continuously under bright lights	• Keep side rails up. • Provide baby with non-flammable toys only. • Avoid leaving small objects within reach including toys that could cause choking. • Patient feels safe when cuddled and supported. • Transport in size appropriate means (bassinet, stroller, crib). • Inform and discuss with caregiver the importance of using car seat when traveling.
NEONATAL **6-12 Months**	• Introduce yourself to caregiver. • Talk slowly and calmly to infant. • Try to initiate eye contact with infant, but do not force.	• Keep patient warm and dry. • Allow for usual feeding schedule. • Allow familiar caregiver close by. • Allow infant to keep pacifier, blanket or comfort toy.	• Infant has stranger anxiety. • Do not separate from caregiver unless absolutely necessary. • Transport in as small as possible means: crib, stroller, or wagon with side rails. • Keep side rails up. • Provide baby with non-flammable toys only. • Avoid leaving small objects within reach including toys that could cause choking. • Inform and discuss with caregiver the importance of using car seat when traveling.
PEDIATRIC & ADOLESCENT **13-36 Months**	• Introduce yourself. • Self-centered thinking. Patient can understand simple commands and may choose to cooperate. • Do not rush patient. Needs time to think about what has been asked of him. • Allow to touch equipment. • Ask parent to explain directions to child in familiar words.	• Keep patient warm if not active. • Do not separate child from favorite pacifier, blanket, comfort toy, or adult.	• Can tolerate short separation from parent. • Do not leave unsupervised; child does not recognize danger. • Clumsy. Trips easily. • Transport in crib, stroller or wagon with side rails. • Keep side rails up. • Provide baby with non-flammable toys only. • Avoid leaving small objects within reach including toys that could cause choking. • Inform and discuss with caregiver the importance of using car seat when traveling.
PEDIATRIC & ADOLESCENT **3-5 Years**	• Introduce yourself. • Talk to child in simple language. Let child explore and touch equipment. • Since child has imagination, use familiar characters in conversation and explanation (ie., Sesame Street, Disney, Barney). • Include parent in explanations. • If shy or frightened may accept explanations and exams given on "Teddy" or other toy.	• Allow familiar things or faces nearby. • Allow child to talk and verbalize fears.	• Can tolerate some separation from parent. • Able to recognize danger and obey simple commands (in most cases). • Cannot yet understand reasons as to why something is acceptable or unacceptable. • Needs close supervision. • Transport in crib, wagon, or on cart with side rails. • Keep side rails up. • Inform and discuss with caregiver the importance of using car seat when traveling.
PEDIATRIC & ADOLESCENT **6-12 Years**	• Introduce yourself. • Able to understand more complex explanations. • Talk to child directly. Allow time for questions. • Still likes to explore equipment before use. • Likes to get involved and make decisions.	• Be subtle in encouraging child to keep comfort object with him. • May need parent. • Use calm, unrushed approach. Allow time for repeated questions. • Permit child some input on decisions.	• Curious. • Able to accept limits. • Transport in wheelchair or on cart with side rails. • Inform and discuss with caregiver and child the importance of using car seat when traveling.
PEDIATRIC & ADOLESCENT **13-17 Years**	• Introduce yourself. • Use adult vocabulary. Do not "talk down" to youth. • Very curious. • Allow time for questions. • Needs privacy.	• Maintain privacy. Is very modest. • Take time for explanations. • Sometimes is comfortable knowing that parent is close by. • Permit adult to accompany youth if desired.	• Starting to be independent. • Can recognize danger. • Transport as an adult. • Inform and discuss with patient the importance of using car seat when traveling.

		Communication	Comfort	Safety
ADULT	**18-65 Years**	• Introduce yourself. • Call patient by title and last name unless patient asks to be called by another name. • Do not address patients with honey, sweetie, dear, etc. • Explain procedures to patient. Give details. • Allow time for questions. • Be respectful.	• Maintain patient's adult privileges; decision-making, privacy, routine of personal habits as much as hospital policy permits. • Offer assistance with personal care. • Inform of available services such as newspapers, coffee, mail, etc. • Inform of hospital/departmental policies such as no smoking, visiting hours, phones.	• Patient's present condition may place patient at risk for falling. May need to use fall precautions. • Keep equipment, cords, supplies, and linen out of patient's path. • Maintain well-lit area. Use night lights if patient desires. • Supply with walking aids if used at home (cane, walker, crutches). Keep these within patient's reach. • Transport using wheelchair or cart with side rails. Weak or confused patients or patients in danger of falling may need safety belt or restraint during transport. Check with patient's nurse to plan for safe transport. • Inform and discuss with patient the importance of using car seat belt when traveling.
GERIATRICS	**65+ Years**	The elderly are a diverse population, whose functional levels vary dramatically within the age group. The following interventions are dependent on individual need. • Introduce yourself. • Do not rush patient. • Talk to patient respectfully. • Call patient by title and last name unless patient asks to be called by another name. • Do not address patients with honey, sweetie, dear, etc. **Hearing:** • Determine if patient uses hearing aid. • Make sure hearing aid is worn. • Check batteries periodically. • Speak slowly and clearly, looking at the patient while you speak. • Do not stand in front of the light source when talking with patient. • Use a deeper voice. Do not shout at the patient. • Patient may need pencil and paper to communicate messages. • Give step by step explanations and instructions as needed.	• Maintain patient's adult privileges: decision-making, privacy, routine of personal habits as much as hospital policy permits. • Offer assistance with personal care. • Inform of available services such as newspapers, coffee, mail, etc. • Inform of hospital/departmental policies such as no smoking, visiting hours, phones. • Do not rush patient. • Help patient to and from the bathroom and in the bathroom if necessary. • Follow home or nursing home habits as much as hospital policy permits. • Tell confused patients who you are, where they are and what time of day it is every time you meet them. If patient is confused, do not try to correct them or argue with patient. • Ask family to bring familiar objects to keep at bedside (robe, blanket, pictures). • Keep patient warm. May need extra sheet or blanket. • Keep water cup, tissue, call light, etc. within reach. • Ask if tap or ice water is preferred.	• Do not rush patient. • Find out if patient is at risk for falls. If yes, refer to falls precautions. • Keep equipment, cords, supplies, and linen out of patient's path. • Determine if patient uses an aid at home (cane, walker, crutches, etc.) When walking, keep these within patient's reach. • Weak and/or confused patients may need frequent reminders to remain seated. • May need repeated offers of assistance with any needs (personal needs included). • Maintain well-lit area. Use night lights. **Vision:** • Put objects where patient can see them. • Determine if patient wears glasses. • Offer to clean patient's glasses. • Have patient wear glasses while awake. • Use caution with temperature of fluids, bath water, heating pads or other equipment. • Transport using wheelchair or cart with side rails. • Weak or confused patients or patients in danger of falling may need safety belt or restraint during transport. Check with patient's nurse to plan for safe transport.

Figure 1.1 Age-specific care considerations. Courtesy St. Joseph Mercy Hospital, Ann Arbor, Michigan. Used with permission.

TABLE 1.2 APPROPRIATE CAREGIVER BEHAVIORS FOR VARIOUS AGE GROUPS

Infant: Birth–1 Year	Toddler: 1–2 Years	Preschool: 2–5 Years	School-Age Child: 5–12 Years
Keep child with parent(s). Use parents to comfort rather than restrain child during hurtful or scary experiences. Explain procedures to parents so they can calm patient. Keep small objects (such as IV tube caps and safety pins) out of child's reach. Ensure that the side of the bed is up. Place visually interesting objects where child can observe them. Provide age- and disease-appropriate toys.	Keep child with parent(s). Use parents to comfort rather than restrain child during hurtful or scary experiences. Explain procedures to parents so they can calm patient. Keep small objects (such as IV tube caps) out of child's reach. Ensure that the side of the bed is up. Toddlers are accustomed to being "on the go." Efforts to interfere with their movements may provoke negative displays, obstinacy, even temper tantrums. Interact with children on their terms, which may mean moving about with them.	Keep child with parent(s). Use parents to comfort rather than restrain child during hurtful or scary experiences. Explain procedures in simple words, describing only what patients will see, what things will look like outside the body. For example, if child will have an IV, demonstrate the tubing and IV needle hub. Don't show or talk about things that will not be visible to the child, such as the needle. Provide activities that engage the child and lessen anxiety when appropriate.	Allow independent movement as appropriate. Explain procedures in greater detail. Offer choices, when possible, to allow children to experience some control over their bodies and environment. For example, ask if patient would like you to make the bed now or after breakfast. Explain how long a painful procedure will take. This will avoid or shorten the child's attempts to stall the experience. When possible, give a tour before hospitalization to acquaint child with the environment.

Adolescent: 12–18 Years	Young Adult: 18–40 Years	Middle Adult: 40–65 Years	Older Adult: 65+ Years
Show interest in visits by the patient's peers, supporting and complimenting positive behavior. Involve adolescents fully in decisions about their health care. Express interest in and support adolescents who exhibit concern about scars or imperfections, even if they are minor. Body image is very important at this age.	Involve patient in decision making about all aspects of health care. Review with patient what treatments are scheduled, including when they will take place, and so on. Knowing what to expect next helps the patient adapt to unfamiliar surroundings and routines. Listen to patient's concerns about the effect illness will have on progress toward lifelong goals like meaningful relationships, offspring, and employment.	Involve patient in decision making about all aspects of health care. Ask if patient would like a family member or other person present to provide support, help with hearing and clarifying information when needed, or making a health care decision. Provide information when the family member or other person arrives. Review with patient what treatments are scheduled, including when they will take place, and so on. Knowing what to expect next helps the patient adapt to unfamiliar surroundings and routines.	Ask patient about the routine followed at home, and adapt the hospital routine as much as possible to the patient's at-home routine. Review with patient what treatments are scheduled, including when they will take place, and so on. Knowing what to expect next helps the patient adapt to unfamiliar surroundings and routines. Ask if patient would like a family member present to provide support in making a health care decision. Provide information needed when the family member arrives.

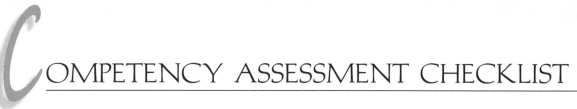

COMPETENCY ASSESSMENT CHECKLIST

Neonatal and Pediatric Care

Name: _____ Date Completed: _____

Activity	Needs Improvement	Date Met	Initials	Comments
1. Demonstrates the ability to assist a breast-feeding mother				
2. Uses correct infant bottle-feeding method				
3. Diapers a baby and provides skin care				
4. Performs infant bath and skin assessment				
5. Demonstrates proper procedure for measuring vital signs in an infant				
6. Provides age-appropriate toys and a safe environment				
7. Communicates with child using language appropriate for age				
8. Comforts a small preschool child in pain				
9. Includes parent in the plan of care				
10. Correctly identifies growth and development stages of infants, toddlers, preschoolers, school-age children, and adolescents				
11. Correctly measures infant's head circumference				
12. Recognizes the impact of illness on children and anticipates that they may behave at a lower developmental level while sick				
13. Anticipates teenager's need for independence and involvement in the plan of care				

COMPETENCY ASSESSMENT CHECKLIST

Older Adult Care

Name: _____ Date Completed: _____

_____

Activity	Needs Improvement	Date Met	Initials	Comments
1. Attends unit education program and/or completes module				
2. *Initial Assessment:* a. Consistently uses geriatric assessment tools (Admission Assessment, Nutrition Screening Tool) in obtaining admission/baseline data for Functional Area Guidelines b. Implements strategies of either maintenance or restoration				
3. *Ongoing Assessment:* a. Identifies when patient demonstrates change in status, revises plan of care collaboratively with interdisciplinary team, communicates change in care (care plan, board, report sheet)				
4. *Patient Education:* a. Collaborates with interdisciplinary team to identify learning needs, provides patient education, and prepares patient for discharge				
5. Demonstrates knowledge and understanding of the physio/psycho/sociological changes of aging, risk factors for iatrogenic illnesses/disorders, and factors that promote optimal functioning and well-being				
a. ***Activity:*** Implements strategies to assist patient to maintain or improve prehospitalization activity level *Examples:* • Evaluates activity orders daily and progress as indicated to increase endurance • Promotes safe environment for ambulation (encourages use of hard-sole shoes/appropriate footware, removes or minimizes physical barriers in room or hall)				

Activity	Needs Improvement	Date Met	Initials	Comments
• Provides assistance and demonstrates proper use of assistive devices for ambulation (gait belt, walker, cane) • Coordinates time in chair with meals when patient is able to tolerate only short periods of time out of bed • Ensures activity plan as written on report sheet and board in patient room				
b. *Cognition:* Implements strategies to promote optimal cognitive functioning *Examples:* • Assesses cognitive status daily (orientation and recall) • Implements strategies to decrease the risk of developing acute confusion (orientation of objects in room, such as clock, calendar, personal objects; maximize sensory input with use of glasses, dentures, hearing aids; use of night light; removal of excess clutter in room) • Monitors use and response to hypnotics, sedatives, and tranquilizers collaboratively with interdisciplinary team • Communicates using techniques that encourage orientation (short, simple phrases spoken slowly, one direction at a time; reality-orientation cues in conversation)				
c. *Depression:* Implements strategies to help patient achieve optimal level of emotional well-being *Example:* • Assesses emotional status and symptoms of depression regularly; initiates referrals to mental health resources for further assessment if necessary				
d. *Elimination:* *Bladder:* Implements strategies to help patient achieve urinary bladder functioning *Examples:* • Provides adequate fluid intake, toileting at regular intervals, path to bathroom well lit and free of clutter, call light within reach • When used, assesses need for Foley on daily basis; recommends removal as soon as possible				

Activity	Needs Improvement	Date Met	Initials	Comments
• Instructs patient on diuretic the effect of some foods and beverages as outlined in Bladder Irritants handout *Bowel:* Implements strategies to help patient achieve optimal bowel functioning *Examples:* • Continues home regimen as appropriate; ensures adequate fluid intake, fiber in diet, and ambulation; allows for uninterrupted time after meals to encourage bowel movement • Implements Bowel Protocol				
e. **Nutrition:** Implements strategies for nutritionally balanced diet and maintenance of admission weight *Examples:* • Performs or encourages oral care before meals; offers fluid or snack between meals; encourages patient to sit in chair for meals and for 30–60 minutes after; assists with menu selection; assists with feeding				
f. **Skin:** Implements strategies to maintain skin integrity, manage pressure, and promote wound healing *Examples:* • Demonstrates and ensures use of polymer pads for incontinence • Demonstrates and ensures use of pressure-reduction devices (blue air cushion, consult CM for specialty bed) • Demonstrates lifting, turning, and body alignment techniques that maintain skin integrity, manage pressure, avoid shearing • Uses skin care techniques that prevent drying (shower versus bed bath, emollients)				
6. Demonstrates awareness of unit **Restraint Philosophy** by applying restraints as last resort or short-term strategy to maintain safety, using least restrictive device needed (mittens, waist belt); reevaluates need daily, and implements **policy fully**				

Source: Chart courtesy St. Joseph Mercy Hospital, Ann Arbor, Michigan. Used with permission.

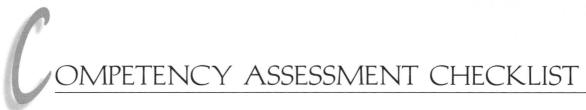

COMPETENCY ASSESSMENT CHECKLIST

Age-Specific Criteria

Name: _____ Date Completed: _____

RN Compentency	Adolescent 14–17 Years	Adult 18–64 Years	Geriatrics 65+ Years	Date Met/ Signature
1a. *Patient Care:* Collects data utilizing age-appropriate technique, tool, or equipment	On admission utilizes the peds assessment tool or reviews the peds assessment information	Assesses functional health patterns on admission	On admission, assesses/reviews sensory information and identifies sensory deficits (e.g., hearing impairments)	Adolescent: ____ _____ Adult: _____ _____ Geriatric: _____ _____
1b. *Patient Care:* Interprets data and modifies care appropriate to age of the patient	Utilizes knowledge of growth and development when planning nursing care interventions	Demonstrates knowledge and use of assistive devices: walker, canes, BSC; teaches hemi technique	Plan of care identifies interventions to maintain skin integrity (*prn*) Drug therapy alteration (narcotics, Torodol)	Adolescent: ____ _____ Adult: _____ _____ Geriatric: _____ _____
2. Uses communication techniques appropriate for the age of the patient	Demonstrates an understanding of adolescent behaviors/needs by allowing choices or by setting limits	Demonstrates active listening skills, allowing time for patient to ask questions	Allows time for patient to process information and allows time for patient to respond	Adolescent: ____ _____ Adult: _____ _____ Geriatric: _____ _____
PCA/PCT Compentency	**Adolescent 14–17 Years**	**Adult 18–65 Years**	**Geriatrics 65+ Years**	**Date Met/ Signature**
1. *Patient Care:* Collects data utilizing age-appropriate technique, tool, or equipment	Uses tympanic thermometer when cognitive level or behaviors dictate	Uses correct size B/P cuff as needed	Maintains turning schedule to prevent skin breakdown and reports observations to the RN	Adolescent: ____ _____ Adult: _____ _____ Geriatric: _____ _____
2. Uses communication techniques appropriate to the age of the patient	Calls patient by name preferred, recognizing the need to establish an identity at this stage of development	Calls patient by name preferred	Establishes that patient is wearing glasses, hearing aids, or has memory log (e.g., tools needed for effective communication)	Adolescent: ____ _____ Adult: _____ _____ Geriatric: _____ _____

RN/Preceptor must observe behaviors and sign appropriate section.

CHAPTER 2
STANDARD PRECAUTIONS, ASEPSIS, AND STERILE TECHNIQUE

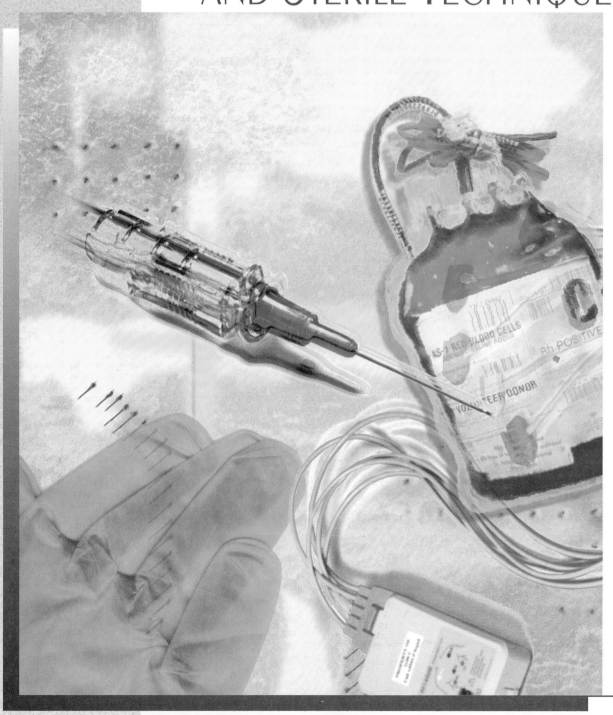

INTRODUCTION

*C*aregivers who work in a health care environment need to understand disease transmission and how to reduce the spread of infection. The Centers for Disease Control and Prevention (CDC) have updated and expanded their guidelines for the protection of employees in health care settings. The CDC's expanded guidelines consist of two tiers of precautions: Standard Precautions and Transmission-based precautions. This chapter reviews the relationship between these precautions and isolation and universal precautions. The procedures for handwashing and the proper use of protective equipment are described. The guide to OSHA compliance regarding blood-borne infections includes the value of Hepatitis B vaccine immunization to reduce occupational risk. Competency assessment for infection control and sterile technique can serve as a foundation to protect both caregivers and patients.

This chapter prepares caregivers to do the following:

1. Describe compliance with Standard Precautions.

2. List indications for airborne, droplet, and contact precautions.

3. Identify the OSHA-required elements of an exposure control plan to avoid blood-borne pathogen infections.

4. Differentiate clean and sterile techniques.

5. Demonstrate the procedure for handwashing.

6. Demonstrate putting on a gown, mask, and sterile gloves.

7. Open a sterile package.

Key Terms

Asepsis The absence of microorganisms (germs).

Aseptic Germfree, without disease-producing organisms.

Autoclave Device used to achieve sterility of an item through heat, pressure, and steam.

Bacteria Unicellular microorganism.

Disinfection The process of destroying as many pathogenic microorganisms as possible from inanimate objects.

Hepatitis B Blood-borne disease, affects the liver, easily transmitted within the health care setting following parenteral exposure.

Infections Due to a pathogen producing a reaction that may cause soreness, tenderness, redness, and/or pus, fever, change in drainage, and so on.

Microorganism A living thing that is so small it cannot be seen with the naked eye but only through a microscope.

Nosocomial Infection Hospital-acquired infection.

Pathogen Disease-producing microorganism.

Sterilization The process of killing all microorganisms, including spores.

Virus A type of microorganism much smaller than bacteria; can survive only in other living cells.

Overview of Standard Precautions

Isolation Precautions

As hospitals continue to collect data and analyze trends in the frequency of pathologens, it has become apparent that specific disease entities require additional precautions over and above the *universal precautions* in order to interrupt disease transmission. Universal precautions centered around this concept: Treat all body fluids as if infectious. Additional categories of precautions were added to interrupt increasingly prevalent conditions that were transmitted through the contact, droplet, or airborne route. The Centers for Disease Control and Prevention (CDC) has established two-tier precaution guidelines consisting of (1) Standard Precautions, which incorporate the concepts behind the universal precautions, and (2) transmission-based precautions, which use Standard Precautions plus additional prevention methods to prevent the spread of disease through the contact, droplet, and airborne routes.

Most hospitals have chosen to follow the CDC guidelines exactly. Some hospitals have isolation policies that are similar in underlying principle but have different details. The basic components of every isolation program should include the following:

- *Specific policies for caregivers to follow with all patients to protect against the transmission of disease.* Precautions are used as a safeguard and must be followed regardless of whether a patient has been diagnosed with an infectious disease. All body fluids are considered infectious—including blood, urine, and saliva—and a barrier is worn to prevent the caregiver from coming into contact with the moist body substance.

- *An isolation policy to prevent the transmission of infectious diseases that are spread on air currents.* These policies are often called "airborne precautions" and may include placing the patient in a specific room with a unique airflow pattern.

- *Established methods for the safe handling of "sharps" to prevent injuries and deep exposure to body fluids.*

Standard Precautions

Isolation precautions are designed to reduce the risk of exposure to microorganisms and to prevent the spread of infectious disease. Standard Precautions, the main component of all isolation precautions, are necessary for the safety of caregivers and patients. Standard Precautions assist in controlling the spread of nosocomial infections, which are hospital-acquired infections.

Standard Precautions apply to all of the following:

- Blood
- All body fluids—secretions and excretions—except sweat, whether or not they contain visible blood
- Nonintact skin
- Mucous membranes

To comply with these precautions, caregivers must wear personal protective equipment in addition to following the appropriate practice. The chart at the top of page 21 explains some of the specifics.

Caregivers adhere to Standard Precautions when delivering care to all patients. Table 2.1 identifies the selected procedures or patient interactions for which Standard Precautions are necessary and indicates the specific precautions or equipment to be used.

STANDARD PRECAUTIONS

- *Gloves:* Must be worn during procedures or situations in which there is or might be exposure to blood, body fluids, secretions, and excretions (except sweat), regardless of whether they contain visible blood, nonintact skin, or mucous membranes.

- *Gown or apron:* Must be worn during procedures or situations in which there might be exposure to body fluids, blood, draining wounds, or mucous membranes.

- *Mask and protective eyewear (face shield):* Must be worn during procedures that are likely to generate droplets of body fluids or blood or when the patient is coughing excessively.

- *Handwashing:* Hands must be washed before gloving and after gloves are removed. Hands and other skin surfaces must be washed immediately and thoroughly if contaminated with body fluids or blood, after all patient care activities, and after gloves are removed. Caregivers who have open cuts, sores, or dermatitis on their hands must wear gloves for all patient contact or be removed from patient contact until their hands have healed.

- *Transportation:* When transporting any patient, ensure that precautions are maintained to minimize the risk of transmission of microorganisms to other patients and contamination of environmental surfaces or equipment.

- *Multiple-use patient care equipment:* When using common equipment or items (for example, a stethoscope or blood pressure cuff) it must be adequately cleaned or disinfected after use or whenever it becomes soiled with blood or other body fluids.

TABLE 2.1 STANDARD PRECAUTIONS REQUIRED FOR SELECTED PROCEDURES

Procedure	Handwashing	Gloves	Gown	Mask	Eyewear
Talking to patient					
Obtaining patient's blood pressure	×				
Performing any procedure in which hands have potential to or become soiled with blood/body fluids	×	×			
Examining patient without touching blood/body fluids or mucous membranes	×	×			
Touching blood/body fluids, mucous membranes broken skin, lesions, or contaminated equipment	×	×			
Drawing blood	×	×			
Doing heel stick	×	×			
Inserting an intravenous catheter	×	×			
Between patient contact	×				
Suctioning a patient's respiratory tract	×	× ⟶ *Note:* Use gown, mask and eyewear if blood/body fluid exposure is likely.			
Handling soiled waste, linen, and other materials	×	× ⟶ *Note:* Use gown if waste or linen is saturated and may soil your clothing.			
Participating in operative and other procedures that produce splattering or spraying of blood/body fluids	×	×	×	×	×

Transmission-Based Precautions

The second component or tier of the isolation system consists of the transmission-based precautions. These are designed to be used with patients documented or suspected to be infected or colonized with a highly transmissible pathogen for which additional precautions beyond standard precautions are needed to interrupt disease transmission. There are three types of transmission-based precautions: contact, droplet, and airborne precautions.

CONTACT PRECAUTIONS

Visitors report to nursing station before entering the room.

- *Indications:* For patients infected with a microorganism that is not easily treated with antibiotics, such as *Clostridium difficile, Shigella,* respiratory syncytial virus, herpes, and impetigo.
- *Patient placement:* Private room (if not available, place patient with another patient with similar microorganism but no other infection).
- *Gloves:* Wear gloves when entering the room and for all contact with patient and patient items, equipment, and body fluids.
- *Gown:* Wear a gown when entering the room if you anticipate that your clothing will have substantial contact with the patient, environmental surfaces, or items in the patient's room.
- *Mask and eyewear:* These are indicated if potential exists for exposure to infectious body material.
- *Handwashing:* Wash hands after removing gloves, and ensure that hands do not touch potentially contaminated environmental surfaces or items in the patient's room.
- *Transportation:* Limit the movement and transportation of the patient from the room.
- *Patient care equipment:* When possible, dedicate the use of noncritical patient care equipment to a single patient. Reusable equipment must be adequately cleaned or disinfected upon removal from a patient's room or between patient uses.

Always use Standard Precautions.

DROPLET PRECAUTIONS

Visitors report to nursing station before entering the room.

- *Indications:* For patients infected with microorganisms that are transmitted by droplets and can be generated by the patient during coughing, such as invasive *Haemophilus* influenza, *Neisseria* meningitidis, influenza, and diphtheria.
- *Patient placement:* Private room (if not available, place patient with another patient who has an active infection with the same microorganism).
- *Gloves:* Gloves must be worn when in contact with blood and body fluids.
- *Gowns:* A gown must be worn during procedures or situations in which there will be exposure to body fluids, blood, draining wounds, or mucous membranes.
- *Mask and eyewear:* In addition to the Standard Precautions, wear a mask when working within three feet of patient (or when entering patient's room).
- *Handwashing:* Hands must be washed before gloving and after gloves are removed.
- *Transportation:* Limit the movement and transportation of the patient from the room. If necessary to move the patient, minimize dispersal of droplets by masking the patient if possible.
- *Patient care equipment:* When patient care equipment or items are shared, they must be adequately cleaned or disinfected.

Always use Standard Precautions.

AIRBORNE PRECAUTIONS

Visitors report to nursing station before entering the room.

- *Indications:* For patients known or suspected to be infected with microorganisms transmitted by airborne droplet nuclei that remain suspended in the air, such as tuberculosis, chicken pox, and measles.
- *Patient placement:* Private room with negative air pressure in relation to the surrounding areas. Keep doors closed at all times.
- *Gloves:* Same as Standard Precautions.
- *Gown or apron:* Same as Standard Precautions.
- *Mask and eyewear:* For known or suspected pulmonary tuberculosis, the N-95 (respirator) mask must be worn by all individuals before entering room. For known or suspected airborne viral disease (for example, chickenpox or measles), standard mask should be worn by anyone entering the room who is susceptible to the disease. When possible, those who are susceptible should not enter the room.
- *Handwashing:* Hands must be washed before and after gloves are removed. Skin surfaces must be washed immediately and thoroughly when contaminated with body fluids or blood.
- *Transportation:* Limit the transportation of the patient from the room. If transportation is necessary, place a mask on the patient if possible.
- *Patient care equipment:* All equipment or items (stethoscope, thermometer) must be adequately cleaned or disinfected before being used with another patient.

Always use Standard Precautions.

Use of Personal Protective Equipment

Review the procedures on pages 24–27 to ensure your proper use of personal protection equipment.

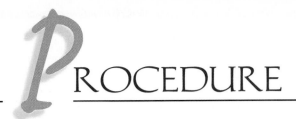

PROCEDURE

Applying a Gown

1. Wash your hands. If you are wearing a long-sleeve garment or uniform, roll your sleeves above your elbows (Figure 2.1).

2. Unfold the isolation gown so that the opening is facing you.

3. Put your arms into the sleeves of the isolation gown.

4. Fit the gown at the neck, making sure your uniform is covered.

5. Reach behind and tie the neck back with a simple shoelace bow, or fasten the adhesive strip.

6. Grasp the edges of the gown and pull them to the back.

7. Overlap the edges of the gown, closing the opening and covering your uniform completely.

8. Tie the waist ties in a bow, or fasten the adhesive strip.

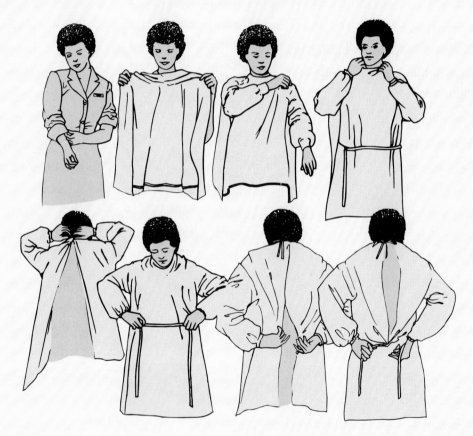

Figure 2.1

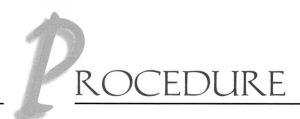

PROCEDURE

Removing a Gown

1. Untie the waist belt or ties (Figure 2.2a).
2. Untie the neck ties, being careful to avoid coming in contact with your neck, or have someone else untie the gown for you (Figure 2.2b).
3. Pull the sleeve off by grasping each shoulder at the neckline (Figure 2.2c).
4. Turn the sleeves inside out as you remove them from your arms (Figure 2.2d).
5. Holding the gown away from your body by the inside of the shoulder seams, fold it inside out, bringing the shoulders together (Figure 2.2e).
6. Roll the gown up with the inside out, and discard (Figure 2.2f).
7. Remove gloves being careful to not contaminate yourself (Figure 2.2g).
8. Remove mask, touching only the strings, and discard (Figure 2.2h).
9. Wash hands (Figure 2.2i).

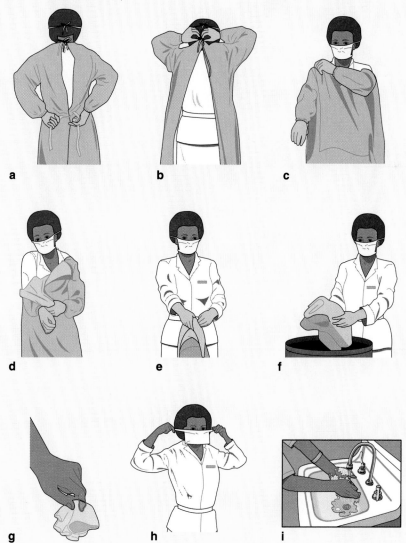

a   b   c

d   e   f

Figure 2.2   g   h   i

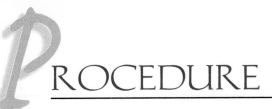

PROCEDURE

Removing Gloves

1. With the gloved fingers of one hand, grasp the glove of the other hand just below the cuff (Figure 2.3a).

2. Turn the glove inside out as you pull it off your hand (Figure 2.3b).

3. Place your ungloved index and middle fingers inside the cuff of the remaining glove (Figure 2.3c).

4. Turning the cuff downward, pull it inside out as you remove your hand (Figure 2.3d).

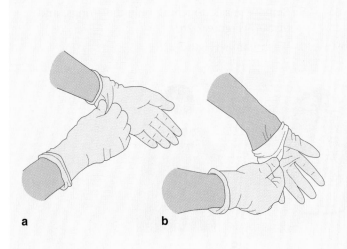

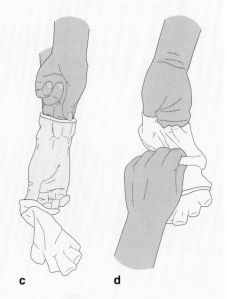

Figure 2.3

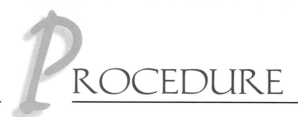

PROCEDURE

Handwashing

1. Assemble your equipment, which should be found at all times at every sink in the health care institution:
   a. Soap
   b. Paper towels
   c. Warm running water
   d. Wastepaper basket
2. Completely wet your hands and wrists under the running water. Keep your fingertips pointed downward.
3. Apply soap.
4. Hold your hands lower than your elbows while washing.
5. Work up a good lather. Spread it over the entire area of your hands and wrists. Get soap under your nails and between your fingers. Wash the back of each hand (Figure 2.4).

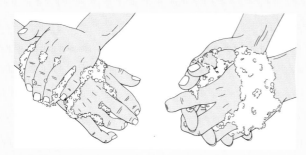

Figure 2.4

6. Clean under your nails by rubbing your nails across the palm of your hand.
7. Use a rotating and rubbing (frictional) motion for 15 seconds:
   a. Rub vigorously.
   b. Rub one hand against the other hand and wrist.
   c. Rub between your fingers by interlacing them.
   d. Rub up and down to reach all skin surfaces on your hands, between your fingers, and 2 inches above your wrists.
   e. Rub the tips of your fingers against your palms to clean with friction around the nail beds.

8. Rinse well. Rinse from 2 inches above your wrists to the hands. Hold your hands and fingertips down under running water (Figure 2.5).

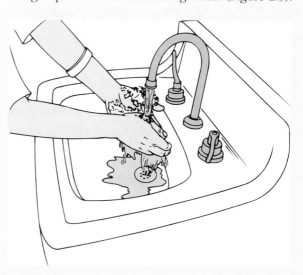

Figure 2.5

9. Dry thoroughly with paper towels.
10. Turn off the faucet, using a paper towel. Never touch the faucet with your hands after washing (Figure 2.6).

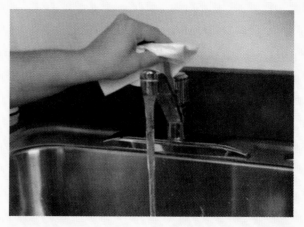

Figure 2.6

11. Discard the paper towel into the wastepaper basket. Do not touch the basket.

Blood-Borne Infections: Guide to OSHA Compliance

All facilities with employees who are subject to exposure of blood-borne pathogens are required to establish a written Exposure Control Plan. This plan must include exposure determination, Standard Precautions, engineering and work practice controls, hepatitis B prophylaxis, training and education, and record keeping:

- *Exposure determination* is defined by OSHA as "any reasonably anticipated skin, eye, mucous membrane or parenteral contact with blood or other potentially infectious materials that may result from the performance of an employee's duties."

- *Standard Precautions* assume that every direct contact with body fluids is potentially infectious. This concept requires that all caregivers or employees who may come into direct contact with body fluids be protected as though such body fluids were infected with hepatitis B or HIV. OSHA emphasizes three major components as part of the Standard Precautions: barrier precautions, handwashing, and sharps precautions.

- *Engineering and work practice controls* are required to reduce the risk of employee exposure to potentially infectious materials.

- *Hepatitis B prophylaxis* is a series of three injections of Hepatitis B vaccine. It must be made available to all employees who could be exposed to blood or other infectious material. Employers are required to pay all costs associated with the hepatitis B immunization program.

- *Training and education programs* must be made available to all employees who may be exposed to blood or other infectious material.

- Records must be kept on hepatitis B vaccination and postexposure follow-up. Records are confidential and maintained for the duration of employment plus 30 years.

Facilities are required to identify all job classifications that involve occupational exposure or risk of exposure to blood and other potentially dangerous body fluids and materials. Training and immunization must be provided to these employees within 10 days of initial assignment to a job that puts the employee at occupational risk.

Asepsis and Sterile Technique

When working in a health care environment, it is important to assist patients to maintain their best possible physical state. To do so, caregivers might be required to practice the principles of asepsis (aseptic technique). When practiced correctly, these standards protect the patient from exposure to germs and help prevent infections.

Asepsis means the absence of microorganisms. Asepsis can be achieved by preventing the conditions that allow pathogens to live, multiply, and spread. As a caregiver, you share the responsibility to prevent the spread of infection by using aseptic, or sterile, technique. (*Aseptic technique* and *sterile technique* are terms that can be used interchangeably. For the rest of this chapter, we will use the term *sterile technique*.)

Sterile technique encompasses the steps followed to prevent contamination by germs. By following these steps very carefully, you will be able to maintain a sterile, or aseptic (germfree), environment in which to do certain tasks.

When practicing sterile technique, keep the following points in mind:

- A sterile field is an area that you create to work from when you are doing a sterile procedure. This area must remain dry in order to remain sterile. You can use a sterile wrap from a package to create this field, or you can use sterile towels supplied as part of a supply kit.

- Only sterile items can be on a sterile field. Sterile items have gone through the process of sterilization, which destroys all living microorganisms. If an unsterile item is placed on the field, the field becomes unsterile. If an unsterile item touches a sterile item, the sterile item becomes unsterile.

- Only the top of a table or the counter of a sterile field is considered to be sterile. Anything hanging over the edge of a sterile field is unsterile. The edges of the sterile field itself (approximately 1 inch into the field) are considered unsterile, so be careful that you do not touch these areas with sterile items.

- Do not cross over your sterile field—that is, unless you are wearing a sterile gown and gloves, do not reach over a sterile field. Microbes may drop from your arms or hands onto the sterile field, making it unsterile.

- Do not turn your back on your sterile field. You do not know what is happening when you cannot see your field. Place the sterile field in a location that will allow you to keep it in sight and do your work efficiently.

- You may not touch the sterile field unless you have sterile gloves on.

- When you have sterile gloves on, your hands must be kept above your waist, in front of your body, and in your sight at all times. You may not touch anything that is not sterile. If you do touch an unsterile item, your gloves become contaminated and must be replaced.

- You may drop sterile items onto a sterile field, but if they touch any unsterile item or the unsterile edge of the field, the sterile item becomes contaminated.

- Anything on your sterile field that absorbs moisture from an unsterile item becomes unsterile. For example, if there is wetness on the table on which you open your sterile package and this wetness soaks into your sterile field, the field becomes contaminated.

Surgical conscience is a term used to describe the way you must act and think when you are working with sterile technique. It is your responsibility to be aware of and maintain your own sterile technique. For example, if no one is around and you contaminate your sterile field, you must be aware of this and start over. This protects the patient from microorganisms and germs that could cause an infection.

It is important to know the difference between clean technique and sterile technique. Some procedures are performed with clean technique. For example, clean technique might be used to change a dressing over a closed surgical wound or to reinforce a dressing. Clean technique involves using clean gloves and clean supplies (they do not need to be sterile, but they may be). You do not need to use sterile technique when doing something "cleanly," but you must still avoid contaminating your clean supplies and clean gloves. Clean items become contaminated if you drop them on the floor; clean gloves become contaminated if you use them to touch something dirty. The registered nurse (RN) will tell you what type of technique (clean or sterile) to use during a procedure.

Following (pages 31–33) are procedures for putting on sterile gloves and for opening a sterile package. These procedures are referred to in many advanced skills but are only described in this chapter.

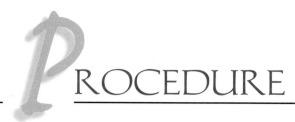

PROCEDURE

Putting on Sterile Gloves

1. Wash hands.
2. Select a pair of wrapped gloves in a size that will fit your hands snugly.
3. Check to be certain that the gloves are sterile:
   a. Package intact, with no signs of dampness?
   b. Seal of sterility?
4. Place the package on a clean, dry, flat surface.
5. Open the wrapper, handling only the outside (Figure 2.7a and b).

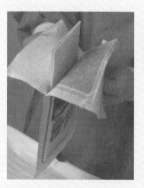 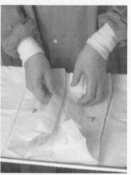

Figure 2.7a   **Figure 2.7b**
Putting on sterile gloves. If either glove tears or becomes contaminated, remove both gloves and start again with a new pair.

6. Use your left hand to pick up the right glove. Touch only the inside folded cuff (Figure 2.7c). *Do not touch the outside of the glove!*

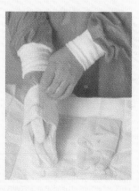

Figure 2.7c

7. Put the glove on your right hand (Figure 2.7d).

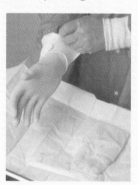

Figure 2.7d

8. Use your gloved right hand to pick up the left glove:
   a. Place the finger of your gloved right hand under the cuff of the left glove (Figure 2.7e).
   b. Lift the glove up and away from the wrapper, and pull it onto your left hand.
   c. Continue pulling left glove up to wrist. Be certain that the gloved right thumb does not touch your skin or clothing (Figure 2.7f).

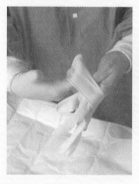 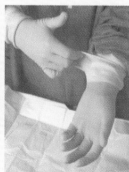

Figure 2.7e   **Figure 2.7f**

9. With your gloved left hand, place fingers under the cuff of the right glove and pull it up over your right wrist.
10. Adjust the fingers of the gloves as necessary.
11. If either glove tears, remove both and begin the procedure again with another pair.

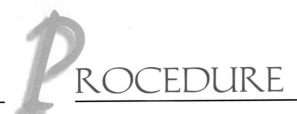

PROCEDURE

Opening a Sterile Package

1. Wash hands.
2. Assemble the equipment and supplies:
   a. Sterile gloves
   b. Sterile package
3. Check to be certain all supplies are sterile:
   a. Package intact, with no signs of dampness?
   b. Seal of sterility?
4. Place the package on a dry, flat, clean work surface (an over-bed table, for example). Position the package so that the first edge to be unfolded will be pulled away from you. (By opening the package away from you with the first motion, you will not have to reach across your sterile area again.) The outer wrap of the package will serve as a sterile field to work on (Figure 2.8a).

5. Slowly pull the corners at the right and left of the package (Figure 2.8b). This exposes the inside of the package.
6. Carefully pull back the corner pointing toward you (Figure 2.8c).
7. If you are going to add sterile items to your field, do so now (Figure 2.9). Remember that the edge (1 inch around) of your sterile field, and anything hanging over the edge of your work area, is contaminated.
8. Do not touch anything inside your sterile package or sterile field until you have put your sterile gloves on.

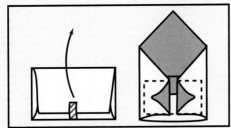

a

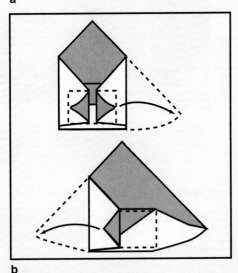

b

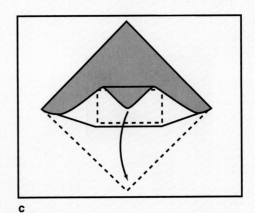

c

Figure 2.8 Opening a sterile package. Always begin opening a sterile package away from you. Never cross over your sterile field with your hands or arms.

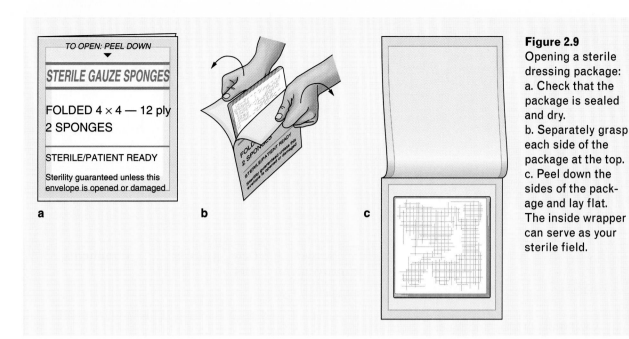

Figure 2.9
Opening a sterile dressing package:
a. Check that the package is sealed and dry.
b. Separately grasp each side of the package at the top.
c. Peel down the sides of the package and lay flat. The inside wrapper can serve as your sterile field.

Asceptic and sterile technique are particularly important in any area where surgical procedures are performed or in an operating room environment. A preceptor will review objectives and performance expectations specific to the procedures that are performed. The assessment sheet on page 35 is an example of how to assess aspesis and sterile technique competencies of a new operating room or same-day surgery facility employees. It is also a useful tool to document progression toward functioning with increasing independence. The caregiver begins oritentation observing and assisting with the room set up, then practices handling instruments and sutures. A preceptor will next coach the orientee through the procedure. Finally the caregiver will be validated or assessed as competent to scrub independently on selected surgical cases.

S U M M A R Y

Standard Precautions, asepsis, and sterile technique are the foundation of all patient care delivery. The risk of infection to yourself or the acquisition of a hospital-acquired nosocomial infection are greatly reduced through following the recommendations and procedures described in this chapter. Handwashing is the most important measure you can take to prevent the spread of microorganisms. All caregivers need to know when and what protective items to use to implement Standard or transmission-based precautions. Following OSHA recommendations and receiving the hepatitis B vaccine are ways to further reduce occupational risks.

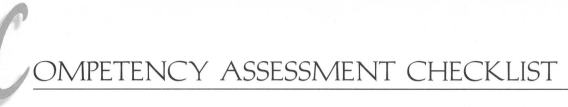

Name: _____ Date Completed: _____

_____

Activity	Needs Improvement	Date Met	Initials	Comments
1. Demonstrates proper handwashing procedure:				
a. Application of soap and water				
b. Use of friction				
c. Use of paper towel to shut off faucets				
2. Demonstrates proper gloving procedure:				
a. Application of nonsterile disposable gloves				
b. Removal of nonsterile disposable gloves				
c. Application of sterile disposable gloves				
d. Removal of sterile disposable gloves				
3. Demonstrates proper gowning procedure:				
a. Application of gown and mask				
b. Removal of gown and mask				
4. Demonstrates proper procedure for opening sterile package				

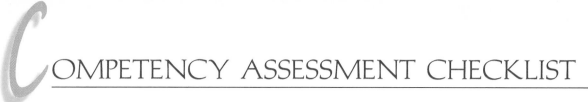

COMPETENCY ASSESSMENT CHECKLIST

Surgical Procedure Orientation Log

Name: _____ Date Completed: _____

_____

Activity	Needs Improvement	Date Met	Initials	Comments
1. Attire is consistent with policy:				
a. Uses splash shield/personnel protective devices appropriately				
2. Demonstrates aseptic technique opening supplies/cases				
a. Always checks external and internal indicators on all supplies opened:				
• Removes container lids and check indicator				
• Checks bottom of container for filter and indicator when removing basket				
3. Demonstrates proper handscrubbing/ gowning/gloving of self and surgical team				
4. Demonstrates beginning understanding/compliance with principles of sterile technique and ability to establish/maintain sterile field and avoid crosscontamination				
5. Demonstrates principles of body substance isolation:				
a. Specimen handling				
b. Room clean up				
6. Demonstrates ability to scrub independently on selected or identified surgical cases or procedures:				
a. Observes and assists with room set-up, practices handling instruments and sutures				
b. Assumes role of scrub with assistance of preceptor who remains scrubbed in and may assist with instruments, passing sutures, or counting				
c. Assumes responsibility for all aspects of the case including checking supplies and set-up with preceptor available for support				
d. Scrubs and circulates independently				

CHAPTER 3
ADVANCED PATIENT CARE SKILLS

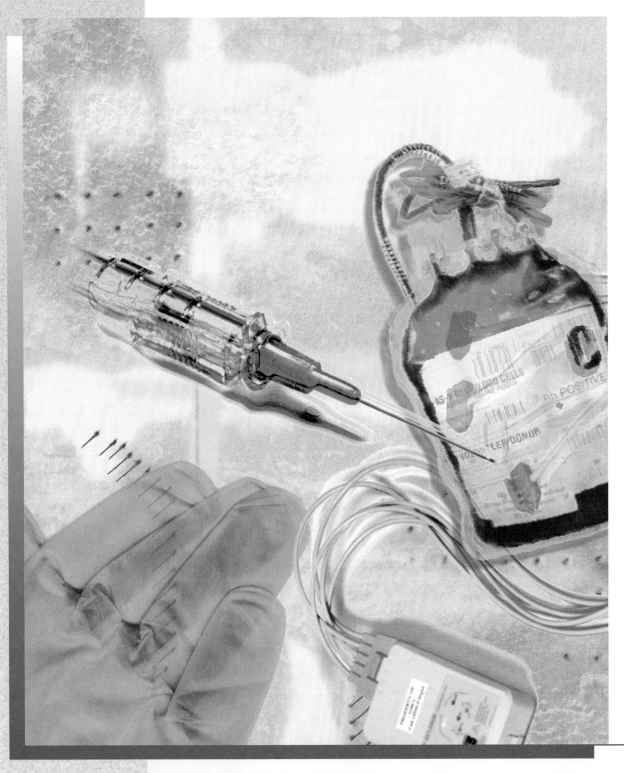

*T*he caregiver needs a broad range of skills and techniques to care for patients and to meet their needs. This chapter includes advanced skills that require knowledge of aseptic technique, knowledge of patients' growth and development needs, and knowledge related to basic anatomy and physiology. These skills generally require physician's orders or are intended to be implemented following an institution's written protocols for care. Each of these skills requires attention to the patient's response to the procedure. Predetermined outcomes or limits require additional skills and intervention by a nurse or physician. Each of these factors will be examined and explained along with the skill.

This chapter prepares caregivers to perform the following skills, which are listed under the relevant section titles:

Clean and Sterile Dressing Changes

Changing a Clean Dressing

Changing an Ostomy Appliance

Changing a Sterile Dressing

Urinary Catheterization

Inserting a Straight Urinary Catheter

Inserting an Indwelling Urinary Catheter

Discontinuing an Indwelling Urinary Catheter

Staple and Suture Removal

Removing Staples

Removing Sutures

Tracheostomy Care

Suctioning a Tracheostomy

Performing Tracheostomy Care (disposable and nondisposable inner cannula)

Performing Tracheostomy Stoma Care

Priming Blood Tubing and Checking Blood Products

Priming Blood Tubing

Checking Blood Products

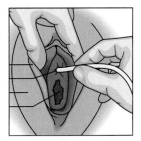
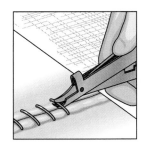
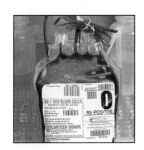

Clean and Sterile Dressing Changes

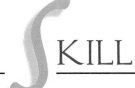

SKILL

Changing a Clean Dressing

Purpose Dressings are placed over and in wounds to facilitate healing. They collect drainage from the wound or incision, help keep the wound clean, and help prevent infection. Dressings may also be used if a patient is not able to look at the wound yet and feels more comfortable seeing it covered. Clean dressings are used when the wound or incision is nearly healed or when there is little risk of infection.

Objectives

The caregiver demonstrates the ability to do the following:

1. Gather the correct supplies.

2. Communicate using a style that reduces the patient's anxiety.

3. Ask the patient about any allergies (latex, tape, etc.).

4. Maintain clean technique.

5. Perform the clean dressing change as delegated.

6. Report the results of the procedure to the RN or preceptor.

Key Terms

Dressing Materials used to cover a wound or incision, including gauze, transparent dressings, and hydrocolloid dressings.

Clean Technique A procedure that is clean but not sterile. Supplies do not need to be sterile but must be clean, not dirty. Clean gloves are worn.

Supplies/Equipment

Dressing materials (as ordered) • Tape • Clean gloves • Biohazard bag or container

Pertinent Points

- A physician's order may be needed for a dressing change. This activity is generally a delegated task, and an RN should be consulted before a dressing is changed.

- A patient may be nervous about having a dressing changed. Explaining the procedure to the patient before beginning may help decrease anxiety.

- Time the dressing change to occur at least 30 minutes after the patient has received pain medication.

Age-Specific Considerations

Certain types of tape used during dressing application may be irritating to the skin of infants, the elderly, or patients with very delicate or thin skin. It may be better to use paper tape with such patients. This tape is not as harsh on fragile skin as other types of tape, and it will help protect the skin from tearing.

*I*t is important to always use clean supplies and clean technique when doing a clean dressing change to promote wound healing without infection. If you think your supplies may not be clean, it is essential to dispose of them and get new supplies.

1. Determine the type, variety, and amount of dressing needed by asking the RN caring for the patient or by checking the physician's order.

2. Gather the supplies.

3. Identify the patient in accordance with institution policy.

4. Explain the procedure to the patient, and ask about any allergies.

5. Wash hands.

6. Position the patient, and ensure privacy.

7. Place the dressing supplies on a clean, dry, flat surface.

8. Put on nonsterile (clean) gloves.

9. Remove, inspect, and document the old dressing. Save it for the RN or preceptor to assess, and then discard it in the biohazard bag or container.

10. Ask the RN or preceptor to inspect the wound.

11. Remove and discard gloves, and put on new nonsterile (clean) gloves.

12. Redress the wound using clean technique, and secure as necessary (Figures 3.1 and 3.2).

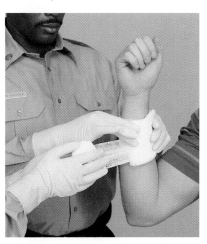
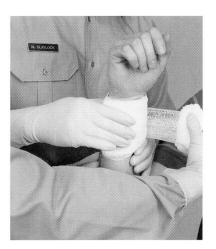

Figure 3.1 Applying a clean dressing using gauze wrap.

13. Discard waste appropriately, remove gloves, and wash hands.

14. Return the patient to a comfortable position.

15. Document the procedure and observations and inform the RN of the completion of the task.

16. Provide input to update the care plan as needed.

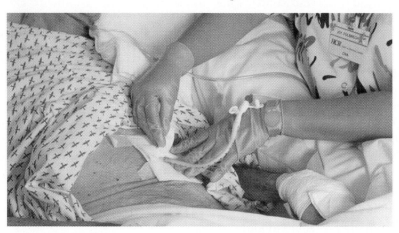

Figure 3.2 Applying a clean dressing to a feeding tube site.

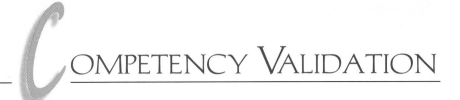

COMPETENCY VALIDATION

Skill: Changing a Clean Dressing

Name _____

Preceptor _____

Date _____

Competency Statement   Changes a clean dressing while demonstrating correct clean technique.

Not Competent: _____ 1. Is <u>unable to state reason</u> for task and <u>needs instructions</u> to perform task.

_____ 2. Understands reason for task but <u>needs instructions</u> to perform task.

Competent: _____ 3. Understands reason for task and is able to perform task but <u>needs to increase speed.</u>

_____ 4. Understands reason for task and is able to perform task <u>proficiently.</u>

Performance Criteria

The caregiver demonstrates the ability to do the following:

_____ 1. Determine the type, variety, and amount of dressing supplies needed by asking the RN caring for the patient or by checking the physician's order.

_____ 2. Gather the supplies.

_____ 3. Identify the patient in accordance with institution policy.

_____ 4. Explain the procedure to the patient, and ask about any allergies.

_____ 5. Wash hands.

_____ 6. Position the patient, and ensure privacy.

_____ 7. Place the dressing supplies on a clean, dry, flat surface.

_____ 8. Put on nonsterile (clean) gloves.

_____ 9. Remove, inspect, and document the old dressing. Save it for the RN or preceptor to assess, and then discard it in the biohazard bag.

_____ 10. Ask the RN or preceptor to inspect the wound.

_____ 11. Remove gloves, and put on new nonsterile (clean) gloves.

_____ 12. Redress the wound using clean technique, and secure as necessary.

_____ 13. Discard waste appropriately, remove gloves, and wash hands.

_____ 14. Return the patient to a comfortable position.

_____ 15. Document the procedure and observations, and inform the RN of the completion of the task.

_____ 16. Provide input to update the care plan as needed.

Advanced Patient Care Skills   CHAPTER 3   *41*

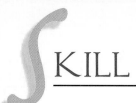

SKILL

Changing an Ostomy Appliance

Purpose Ostomies may be temporary or permanent. An ostomy may be performed to divert the patient's feces from the rectum. Ostomies are often performed when treating diseases such as colon cancer, ulcerative colitis, or Crohn's disease. Feces may be temporarily diverted to allow the bowel to rest and heal after injury. An ostomy may also be performed to divert urine when the bladder or kidneys are injured or diseased.

Objectives

The caregiver demonstrates the ability to do the following:

1. Gather the correct supplies.

2. Communicate using a style that reduces the patient's anxiety.

3. Remove the old ostomy appliance.

4. Note the condition of the patient's skin and stoma.

5. Apply a new appliance.

6. Record the amount of drainage and its consistency and color.

7. Report the results of the procedure to the RN or preceptor.

Key Terms

Ostomy A surgical procedure that creates a new opening, usually in the abdomen, for the discharge of wastes (feces or urine) from the body. Examples include colostomy (feces), ileostomy (feces) and ileoconduit (urine).

Ostomy Appliance A collection pouch that attaches to the skin around the stoma with some type of adhesive.

Stoma A surgically made opening that allows waste to exit the body.

Supplies/ Equipment

Towel • Bed protector • Gloves • Washcloth • Basin of warm water • Wafer with flange (whatever product the patient uses or is supplied in your institution) • New stoma pouch • Stoma adhesive paste

Pertinent Points

- Stomas are usually red due to the large number of blood vessels located in the tissue.

- When giving care to a stoma, it is not uncommon to note a small amount of bleeding. If you note a large amount or if the bleeding does not stop, notify the RN or preceptor immediately.

- Patients react differently to an ostomy. Feelings of loss, fear, anger, and anxiety are normal when adjusting to changes in body image. Allow patients time to express their feelings when you are caring for them.

Age-Specific Considerations

The change in body image that results from an ostomy can be frightening to young children, who may see it as body mutilation. For adolescents and adults, the change can bring out fears and concerns related to sexuality and changes in lifestyle. For elderly patients, an ostomy can generate fears that they may not be able to care for themselves. All of these fears can be addressed through the help of enterostomal therapists (nurses who specialize in the care of ostomy patients) and through support groups where patients can talk with others who have successfully made the transition after an ostomy.

*I*t is crucial to get a good "fit" for the wafer around the patient's stoma. When the fit is poor, feces will irritate the patient's skin and cause it to break down.

1. Wash hands.

2. Explain the procedure to the patient.

3. Provide for privacy.

4. Position the patient for comfort.

5. Expose only the appliance (Figure 3.3). Place a towel over the patient's abdomen and a bed protector under the patient's hips to keep the bed clean.

6. Assemble the equipment, and put on gloves.

7. Gently remove the old pouch and wafer. Measure the contents, and dispose of contents according to institution policy.

8. Wipe the skin around the stoma with a warm, wet washcloth to remove any stool or urine. Rinse the skin carefully. Pat the area dry with a towel. A washcloth can be placed over the stoma to prevent soiling of the area while the new wafer is prepared.

9. Prepare the new wafer by sizing and cutting it to fit over the stoma. The skin should not show between the stoma and the wafer. Use stoma adhesive if necessary (Figure 3.4).

10. Hold the wafer between your hands to warm it and make it more flexible. Apply the new wafer to the skin. Make sure there are no air pockets under the wafer. Hold it in place for 30 seconds to help the adhesive stick well.

11. Apply stoma pouch to the flange on the wafer. Make sure the pouch is correctly sealed (Figure 3.4c).

12. Remove the towel and bed protector. Clean up the area.

13. Wash hands.

14. Document and report the results and the patient's tolerance to the RN or preceptor.

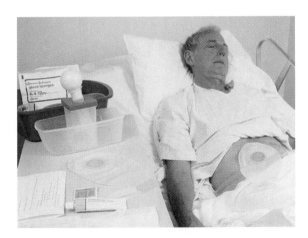

Figure 3.3 Ostomy appliance in place over stoma.

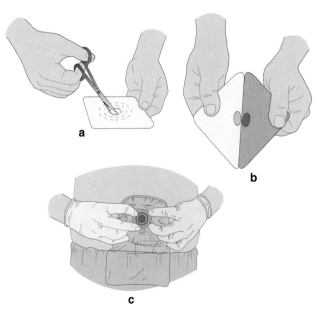

Figure 3.4 Replacing an ostomy appliance.

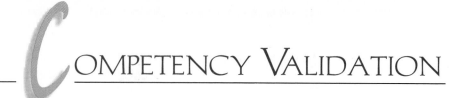

COMPETENCY VALIDATION

Skill: Changing an Ostomy Appliance

Name _____

Preceptor _____

Date _____

Competency Statement

Changes an ostomy appliance while demonstrating correct sterile technique.

Not Competent: _____ 1. Is <u>unable to state reason</u> for task and <u>needs instructions</u> to perform task.

_____ 2. Understands reason for task but <u>needs instructions</u> to perform task.

Competent: _____ 3. Understands reason for task and is able to perform task but <u>needs to increase speed.</u>

_____ 4. Understands reason for task and is able to perform task <u>proficiently.</u>

Performance Criteria

The caregiver demonstrates the ability to do the following:

_____ 1. Wash hands.

_____ 2. Explain the procedure to the patient.

_____ 3. Provide for privacy.

_____ 4. Position the patient for comfort.

_____ 5. Expose only the appliance. Place a towel over the patient's abdomen and a bed protector under the patient's hips to keep the bed clean.

_____ 6. Assemble the equipment, and put on gloves.

_____ 7. Gently remove the old pouch and wafer. Measure the contents, and dispose of contents according to institution policy.

_____ 8. Wipe the skin around the stoma with a warm, wet washcloth to remove any stool or urine. Rinse the skin carefully. Pat the area dry with a towel. A washcloth can be placed over the stoma to prevent soiling of the area while the new wafer is prepared.

_____ 9. Prepare the new wafer by sizing and cutting it to fit over the stoma. The skin should not show between the stoma and the wafer. Use stoma adhesive if necessary.

_____ 10. Hold the wafer between your hands to warm it and make it more flexible. Apply the new wafer to the skin. Make sure there are no air pockets under the wafer. Hold it in place for 30 seconds to help the adhesive stick well.

_____ 11. Apply stoma pouch to the flange of the wafer. Make sure the pouch is correctly sealed.

_____ 12. Remove the towel and bed protector. Clean up the area.

_____ 13. Wash hands.

_____ 14. Document and report the results and the patient's tolerance to the RN or preceptor.

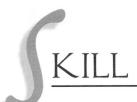

SKILL

Changing a Sterile Dressing

Purpose Dressings are placed over and in wounds to facilitate healing. They collect drainage from the wound or incision, help keep the wound clean, and help prevent infection. Dressings may also be used if a patient is not able to look at the wound yet and feels more comfortable seeing it covered. Sterile dressings are used when wounds or incisions are just beginning to heal or when the risk of infection is high.

The caregiver demonstrates the ability to do the following: Objectives

1. Gather the correct supplies.

2. Communicate using a style that reduces the patient's anxiety.

3. Ask the patient about any allergies (latex, tape, etc.).

4. Maintain sterile technique.

5. Perform the sterile dressing change as delegated.

6. Report the results of the procedure to the RN or preceptor.

Key Terms

Clean Technique A procedure that is clean but not sterile. Supplies do not need to be sterile but must be clean, not dirty. Clean gloves are worn.

Sterile Technique A procedure that remains germfree. Sterile supplies are used, and special steps are taken to ensure that the materials remain sterile. Sterile gloves are worn.

Supplies/ Equipment

Dressing materials (as ordered) • Tape • Clean gloves • Sterile gloves
• Biohazard bag or container

Pertinent Points

• A physician's order may be needed for a dressing change. Generally this activity is a delegated task, and an RN should be consulted before a dressing is changed.

• A patient may be nervous about having a dressing changed.

• Explaining the procedure to the patient before beginning may help decrease anxiety.

• Time the dressing change to occur at least 30 minutes after the patient has received pain medication.

Age-Specific Considerations

Certain types of tape used during dressing application may be irritating to the skin of infants, the elderly, or patients with very delicate or thin skin. It may be better to use paper tape with such patients. This tape is not as harsh on fragile skin as other types of tape, and it will help protect the skin from tearing.

Key Concept

*I*t is important to always use sterile supplies and sterile technique when doing a sterile dressing change to promote wound healing without infection. If you think your supplies may not be sterile, it is essential to dispose of them and get new sterile supplies.

Advanced Patient Care Skills CHAPTER 3   45

1. Determine the type, variety, and amount of dressing needed by asking the RN caring for the patient.

2. Gather the supplies.

3. Identify the patient in accordance with institution policy.

4. Explain the procedure to the patient. Instruct the patient that the procedure will be sterile, and explain the importance of not touching any of the supplies being used. Ask about any allergies.

5. Wash hands.

6. Position the patient and ensure privacy.

7. Place the sterile dressing supplies on a clean, dry, flat surface.

8. Put on nonsterile (clean) gloves.

9. Remove and inspect the old dressing. Save it for the RN or preceptor to assess, and then discard it in the biohazard bag or container.

10. Ask the RN or preceptor to inspect the wound.

11. Remove and discard gloves.

12. Open the sterile dressing supplies, maintaining a sterile field.

13. Put on sterile gloves.

14. Redress the wound using sterile technique, and secure as necessary (Figure 3.5).

15. Discard waste appropriately, remove gloves, and wash hands.

16. Return the patient to a comfortable position.

17. Document the procedure and observations, and inform the RN or preceptor of the completion of the task.

18. Provide input to update the care plan as needed.

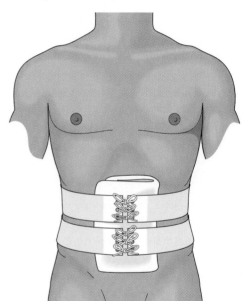

Figure 3.5 A sterile dressing using Montgomery straps.

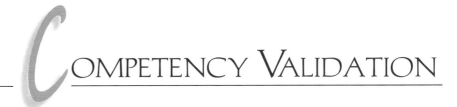

COMPETENCY VALIDATION

Skill: Changing a Sterile Dressing

Name _____

Preceptor _____

Date _____

Competency Statement Changes a sterile dressing while demonstrating correct sterile techniques.

Not Competent: _____ 1. Is <u>unable to state reason</u> for task and <u>needs instructions</u> to perform task.

_____ 2. Understands reason for task but <u>needs instructions</u> to perform task.

Competent: _____ 3. Understands reason for task and is able to perform task but <u>needs to increase speed.</u>

_____ 4. Understands reason for task and is able to perform task <u>proficiently.</u>

Performance Criteria

The caregiver demonstrates the ability to do the following:

_____ 1. Determine the type, variety, and amount of dressing needed by asking the RN caring for the patient or by checking the physician's order.

_____ 2. Gather the supplies.

_____ 3. Identify the patient in accordance with institution policy.

_____ 4. Explain the procedure to the patient. Instruct the patient that the procedure will be sterile, and explain the importance of not touching any of the supplies being used. Ask about any allergies.

_____ 5. Wash hands.

_____ 6. Position the patient, and ensure privacy.

_____ 7. Place the dressing supplies on a clean, dry, flat surface.

_____ 8. Put on nonsterile (clean) gloves.

_____ 9. Remove and inspect the old dressing. Save it for the RN or preceptor to assess, and then discard it in the biohazard bag or container.

_____ 10. Ask the RN or preceptor to inspect the wound.

_____ 11. Remove and discard gloves.

_____ 12. Open the sterile dressing supplies, maintaining a sterile field.

_____ 13. Put on sterile gloves.

_____ 14. Redress the wound using sterile technique, and secure as necessary.

_____ 15. Discard waste appropriately, remove gloves, and wash hands.

_____ 16. Return the patient to a comfortable position.

_____ 17. Document the procedure and observations, and inform the RN or preceptor of the completion of the task.

_____ 18. Provide input to update the care plan as needed.

Urinary Catheterization

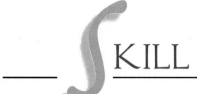

SKILL

Inserting a Straight Urinary Catheter

Purpose Straight catheterization is used to drain the bladder of urine. This procedure is often performed for patients who are experiencing urinary retention or are having difficulty emptying their bladder on their own, for patients who must provide sterile urine samples, or for patients who are undergoing bladder retraining. The catheter is inserted into the bladder, the urine is drained, and then the catheter is removed. This procedure is often performed intermittently.

Objectives

The caregiver demonstrates the ability to do the following:

1. Gather the correct supplies.

2. Communicate using a style that reduces the patient's anxiety.

3. Ask the patient about any allergies (latex, rubber, iodine-based products, tape, etc.).

4. Perform the catheterization.

5. Record the amount of urine obtained.

6. Report the results of the procedure to the RN or preceptor.

Key Terms

Bladder A holding vessel for urine.

Catheterization The process of passing a tubular instrument into a body cavity to insert or remove fluids or gases.

Kidneys The organs that filter the blood to remove waste products and produce urine.

Retention A dangerous condition in which urine becomes trapped in the bladder. Retention can lead to loss of bladder tone, development of renal calculi, and urinary infection.

Ureters Connecting tubes that run between the kidneys and the bladder.

Urethra The normal outlet for urine from the body. The sphincter controls the elimination of urine.

Urinary Meatus The external opening of the urethra.

Supplies/ Equipment

Sterile gloves • Fenestrated drape • Cotton balls • Iodine cleansing solution • Water-soluable lubricant • A size 14–16 French urinary straight catheter • Urine collection basin • Sterile urine cup • Forceps

These items are usually contained within a kit (Figure 3.6).

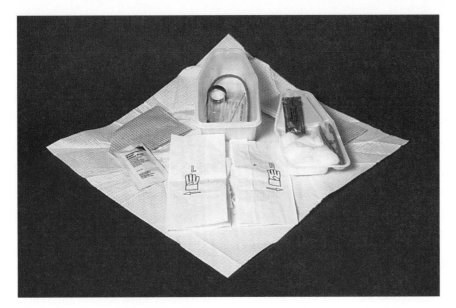

Figure 3.6 Straight catheter kit.

- Urinary catheterization requires a physician's order in most cases.

- Urinary tract infection is the most common complication of being catheterized.

- Although catheterization is a "routine" procedure in health care, it is not routine to patients. They are often hesitant or reluctant about being catheterized. It often helps to relieve the patient's anxiety to explain the purpose of the procedure, provide for privacy, and explain what is happening during the procedure.

- Remove no more than 800 to 1,000 cc of urine at one time to prevent bladder collapse and electrolyte imbalance.

- If the catheter tip is accidentally inserted into the vagina, the catheter is contaminated and must be discarded. The caregiver will need to get a new kit and start over.

Patients of all ages may have concerns and fears about being catheterized. Children may fear where the tube will go inside their body. Elderly patients may fear a loss of mobility and independence. All patients may fear pain and the loss of privacy. To respond to these concerns, be certain to close the door or pull the curtain. Explain the procedure to the patient in terms that he or she can understand; use pictures if appropriate.

*T*he risk of infection increases with the length of time a catheter remains in place. Therefore, whenever appropriate, straight catheterization is preferred over indwelling catheterization because the catheter is removed at the end of the procedure.

Steps for Inserting a Straight Urinary Catheter in a FEMALE Patient

1. Wash hands.

2. Explain the procedure to the patient.

3. Determine if the patient is allergic to iodine-based antiseptics or anything else.

4. Provide for privacy.

5. Position the patient in the dorsal recumbent position with knees flexed, exposing the labia.

6. Drape the patient so that only the perineum is exposed.

7. Assemble the equipment, and put on gloves.

8. Prepare the items in the kit for use during insertion, maintaining clean technique.

9. With nondominant hand, separate the labia minora, and hold this position until the catheter is inserted.

10. Using cotton balls, cleanse the meatus with the iodine cleansing solution:

    a. Making one downward stroke with each cotton ball, begin at the labia on the side farthest from you, and move toward the labia nearest you.

    b. Afterward, wipe once down the center of the meatus.

    c. Wipe once with each cotton ball, and discard. (The forceps may be used to hold the cotton ball.)

11. Direct the open end of the catheter into the collection container. Lubricate and insert the tip of the catheter slowly through the urethral opening 3 to 4 inches or until urine returns.

12. Advance the catheter another .5 to 1.0 inches (Figure 3.7).

13. Allow urine to drain until it stops. Collect a sterile urine specimen if needed. Then remove the catheter slowly, allowing any additional urine to drain.

14. Cleanse the perineal area. Reposition the patient for comfort, and replace the linens.

15. Measure the amount of urine in the collection container, and record.

16. Remove and discard gloves; wash hands.

17. Document and report the results to the RN or preceptor.

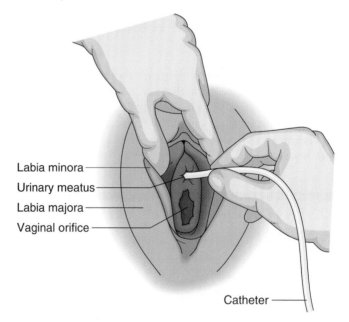

Labia minora
Urinary meatus
Labia majora
Vaginal orifice
Catheter

Figure 3.7 Inserting a urinary catheter in a female patient.

1. Wash hands.

2. Explain the procedure to the patient.

3. Determine if the patient is allergic to iodine-based antiseptics or anything else.

4. Provide for privacy.

5. Drape the patient with bed linens so that only the penis is exposed.

6. Assemble the equipment, and put on gloves.

7. Prepare the items in the kit for use during insertion, maintaining clean technique.

8. Remove the fenestrated drape from the kit, and using nondominant hand, place the penis through the hole in the drape. *Keep dominant hand sterile.*

9. Pull the penis up at a 90-degree angle to the patients's supine body.

10. With nondominant hand, gently grasp the glans (tip) of the penis; retract the foreskin if uncircumcised.

11. Using cotton balls, cleanse the meatus and the glans with the iodine cleansing solution, beginning at the urethral opening and moving toward the shaft of the penis; make one complete circle around the penis with each cotton ball. Direct the open end of the catheter into the collection container.

12. Lubricate and insert the tip of the catheter slowly through the urethral opening 7 to 9 inches or until urine returns (Figure 3.8).

13. Allow urine to drain until it stops. Collect a sterile urine specimen if needed. Then remove the catheter slowly, allowing any additional urine to drain.

14. Cleanse the perineal area, and replace the foreskin of the penis. Reposition the patient for comfort, and replace the linens.

15. Measure the amount of urine in the collection container, and record.

16. Remove and discard gloves; wash hands.

17. Document and report the results to the RN or preceptor.

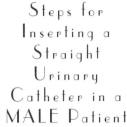

Steps for Inserting a Straight Urinary Catheter in a MALE Patient

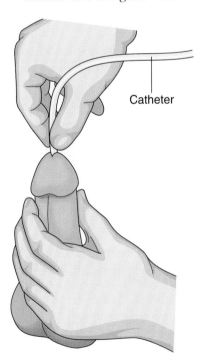

Catheter

Figure 3.8 Inserting a urinary catheter in a male patient.

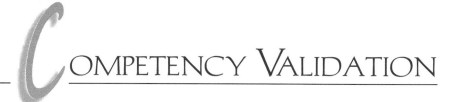
COMPETENCY VALIDATION

Skill: Inserting a Straight Urinary Catheter in a Female Patient

Name _____

Preceptor _____

Date _____

Competency Statement
Inserts a straight urinary catheter in a female patient while demonstrating correct sterile technique.

Not Competent: _____ 1. Is <u>unable to state reason</u> for task and <u>needs instructions</u> to perform task.

_____ 2. Understands reason for task but <u>needs instructions</u> to perform task.

Competent: _____ 3. Understands reason for task and is able to perform task but <u>needs to increase speed.</u>

_____ 4. Understands reason for task and is able to perform task <u>proficiently.</u>

Performance Criteria

The caregiver demonstrates the ability to do the following:

_____ 1. Wash hands.
_____ 2. Explain the procedure to the patient.
_____ 3. Determine if the patient is allergic to iodine-based antiseptics or anything else.
_____ 4. Provide for privacy.
_____ 5. Position the patient in the dorsal recumbent position with knees flexed, exposing the labia.
_____ 6. Drape the patient so that only the perineum is exposed.
_____ 7. Assemble the equipment, and put on gloves.
_____ 8. Prepare the items in the kit for use during insertion, maintaining clean technique.
_____ 9. With nondominant hand, separate the labia minora, and hold this position until the catheter is inserted.
_____ 10. Using cotton balls, cleanse the meatus with the iodine cleansing solution:
    a. Making one downward stroke with each cotton ball, begin at the labia on the side farthest from you, and move toward the labia nearest you.
    b. Afterward, wipe once down the center of the meatus.
    c. Wipe once with each cotton ball, and discard. (The forceps may be used to hold the cotton ball.)
_____ 11. Direct the open end of the catheter into the collection container. Lubricate and insert the tip of the catheter slowly through the urethral opening 3 to 4 inches or until urine returns.
_____ 12. Advance the catheter another 1 to 1.5 inches.
_____ 13. Allow urine to drain until it stops. Collect a sterile urine specimen if needed. Then remove the catheter slowly, allowing any additional urine to drain.
_____ 14. Cleanse the perineal area. Reposition the patient for comfort, and replace the linens.
_____ 15. Measure the amount of urine in the collection container, and record.
_____ 16. Remove and discard gloves; wash hands.
_____ 17. Document and report the results to the RN or preceptor.

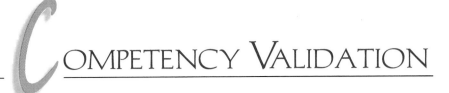

COMPETENCY VALIDATION

Skill: Inserting a Straight Urinary Catheter in a Male Patient

Name _____

Preceptor _____

Date _____

Competency Statement   Inserts a straight urinary catheter in a male patient while demonstrating correct sterile technique.

Not Competent: _____ 1. Is <u>unable to state reason</u> for task and <u>needs instructions</u> to perform task.

_____ 2. Understands reason for task but <u>needs instructions</u> to perform task.

Competent: _____ 3. Understands reason for task and is able to perform task but <u>needs to increase speed.</u>

_____ 4. Understands reason for task and is able to perform task <u>proficiently.</u>

Performance Criteria

The caregiver demonstrates the ability to do the following:

_____ 1. Wash hands.

_____ 2. Explain the procedure to the patient.

_____ 3. Provide for privacy.

_____ 4. Drape the patient with bed linens so that only the penis is exposed.

_____ 5. Assemble the equipment, and put on gloves.

_____ 6. Prepare the items in the kit for use during insertion.

_____ 7. Remove the fenestrated drape from the kit, and using nondominant hand, place the penis through the hole in the drape. Keep dominant hand sterile.

_____ 8. Pull the penis up at a 90-degree angle to the patient's supine body.

_____ 9. With nondominant hand, gently grasp the glans (tip) of the penis; retract the foreskin if uncircumcised.

_____ 10. Using cotton balls, cleanse the meatus and the glans with the iodine cleansing solution, beginning at the urethral opening and moving toward the shaft of the penis; make one complete circle around the penis with each cotton ball. (The forceps may be used to hold the cotton ball.)

_____ 11. Direct the open end of the catheter into the collection container. Lubricate and insert the tip of the catheter slowly through the urethral opening 7 to 9 inches or until urine returns.

_____ 12. Allow urine to drain until it stops. Collect a sterile urine specimen if needed. Then remove the catheter slowly, allowing any additional urine to drain.

_____ 13. Cleanse the perineal area and replace the foreskin of the penis. Reposition the patient for comfort, and replace the linens.

_____ 14. Measure the amount of urine in the collection container, and record.

_____ 15. Remove and discard gloves; wash hands.

_____ 16. Document and report the results to the RN or preceptor.

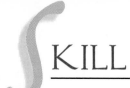

SKILL

Inserting an Indwelling Urinary Catheter

Purpose Urinary catheterization, which involves inserting a hollow catheter up the urethra to the bladder under sterile conditions, is an ancient procedure. Some common reasons to use a catheter are to empty the urine from the bladder, to obtain a urine specimen, to keep the bladder empty (decompression) during certain procedures such as surgery, to instill medications, to bypass an obstruction, and to determine accurate urinary output.

Objectives

The caregiver demonstrates the ability to do the following:

1. Gather the correct supplies.

2. Communicate using a style that reduces the patient's anxiety.

3. Ask the patient about any allergies (latex, rubber, iodine, paper, etc.).

4. Maintain sterile technique.

5. Check the balloon by inflating and deflating it.

6. Perform the catheterization.

7. Record the amount of urine obtained.

8. Report the results of the procedure to the RN or preceptor.

Key Terms

Bladder A holding vessel for urine.

Catheterization The process of passing a tubular instrument into a body cavity to insert or remove fluids or gases.

Kidneys The organs that filter the blood to remove waste products and produce urine.

Retention A dangerous condition in which urine becomes trapped in the bladder. Retention can lead to loss of bladder tone, development of renal calculi, and urinary infection.

Ureters Connecting tubes that run between the kidneys and the bladder.

Urethra The normal outlet for urine from the body. The sphincter controls the elimination of urine.

Supplies/Equipment

Solid drape • Fenestrated drape • Sterile gloves • Urinary catheter • Syringe • Lubricant • Cotton balls • Antiseptic solution • Urine collection tray • Specimen cup • Forceps

These items are usually contained within a kit.

Pertinent Points

- Urinary catheterization requires a physician's order in most cases.
- Although catheterization is a "routine" procedure in health care, it is not routine to patients. They are often hesitant or reluctant about being catheterized. It often helps to relieve the patient's anxiety to explain the purpose of the procedure, provide for privacy, and explain what is happening during the procedure.
- Remove no more than 800 to 1,000 cc of urine at one time to prevent bladder collapse and electrolyte imbalance.

- If the catheter tip is accidentally inserted into the vagina, the catheter is contaminated and must be discarded. The caregiver will need to get a new kit and start over.

Patients of all ages may have concerns and fears about being catheterized. Children may fear where the tube will go inside their body. Elderly patients may fear a loss of mobility and independence. All patients may fear pain and the loss of privacy. To respond to these concerns, be certain to close the door or pull the curtain. Explain the procedure to the patient in terms that he or she can understand; use pictures if appropriate.

*I*nfection is the most common complication of having an indwelling urinary catheter, and the risk of infection increases with the length of time the catheter remains in place. The caregiver's use of correct sterile technique will significantly reduce the patient's risk for infection.

1. Wash hands.
2. Explain the procedure to the patient, emphasizing the need to maintain the sterile field.
3. Determine if the patient is allergic to iodine-based antiseptics or anything else.
4. Provide for privacy.
5. Position the patient in the dorsal recumbent position with knees flexed, exposing the labia.
6. Drape the patient so that only the perineum is exposed.

7. Remove the full drape from the kit with your fingertips, and place, plastic side down, just under the patient's buttocks (ask her to raise her hips).
8. Put on sterile gloves.
9. Prepare the items in the kit for use during insertion, maintaining sterile technique.
10. Test the balloon for defects. Deflate the balloon, and leave the syringe on the catheter (Figure 3.9). Liberally lubricate the catheter tip.

Steps for
Inserting an
Indwelling
Urinary
Catheter in a
Female Patient

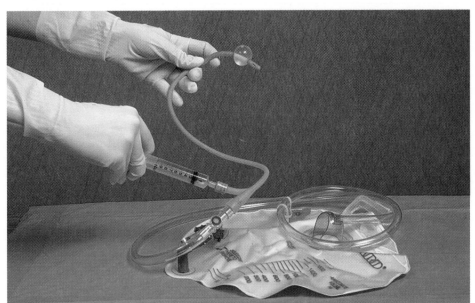

Figure 3.9 Testing the retention balloon of a catheter with a syringe.

11. With nondominant hand, separate the labia minora, and hold this position until the catheter is inserted. (Note: The dominant hand is the only sterile hand now; the contaminated hand continues to separate the labia.) (Forceps may be used to hold the cotton ball.)

12. Using cotton balls, cleanse the meatus with the iodine solution:

    a. Making one downward stroke with each cotton ball, begin at the labia on the side farthest from you, and move toward the labia nearest you.

    b. Afterward, wipe once down the center of the meatus.

    c. Wipe once with each cotton ball, and discard.

13. Insert the tip of the catheter slowly through the urethral opening 3 to 4 inches or until urine returns.

14. Advance the catheter another .5 to 1.0 inches.

15. Inflate the balloon with the attached syringe, and gently pull back on the catheter until it stops, or catches (Figure 3.10). Catch the urine in the collection tray or in the specimen cup (if needed).

16. Measure the amount of urine in the drainage bag, and record.

17. Remove and discard gloves; wash hands.

18. Document and report the results to the RN or preceptor.

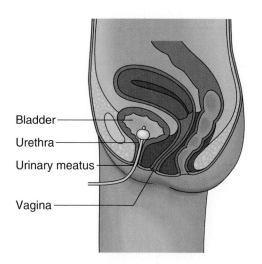

Bladder
Urethra
Urinary meatus
Vagina

Figure 3.10 Side view of female anatomy with indwelling urinary catheter in place.

1. Wash hands.

2. Explain the procedure to the patient.

3. Determine if the patient is allergic to iodine-based antiseptics.

4. Provide for privacy.

5. Assemble the equipment, and put on gloves.

6. Prepare the items in the kit for use during insertion, maintaining sterile technique.

7. Test the balloon for defects. Deflate the balloon, and leave the syringe attached to the catheter (Figure 3.9). Liberally lubricate the catheter tip.

8. Remove the fenestrated drape from the kit, and using nondominant hand, place the penis through the hole in the drape. *Keep dominant hand sterile.*

9. Pull the penis up at a 90-degree angle to the patient's supine body.

10. With nondominant hand, gently grasp the glans (tip) of the penis; retract the foreskin if uncircumcised.

11. Using cotton balls, cleanse the meatus and the glans with iodine solution, beginning at the urethral opening and moving toward the shaft of the penis; make one complete circle around the penis with each cotton ball. (Forceps may be used to hold the cotton ball.)

12. Insert the tip of the catheter slowly through the urethral opening to the bifurcation (Y) of the catheter.

13. Inflate the balloon with the attached syringe, and gently pull back on the catheter until it stops, or catches (Figure 3.11).

14. Replace the foreskin of the penis on uncircumcised males.

15. Measure the amount of urine in the drainage bag, and record.

16. Remove and discard gloves; wash hands.

17. Document and report the results to the RN or preceptor.

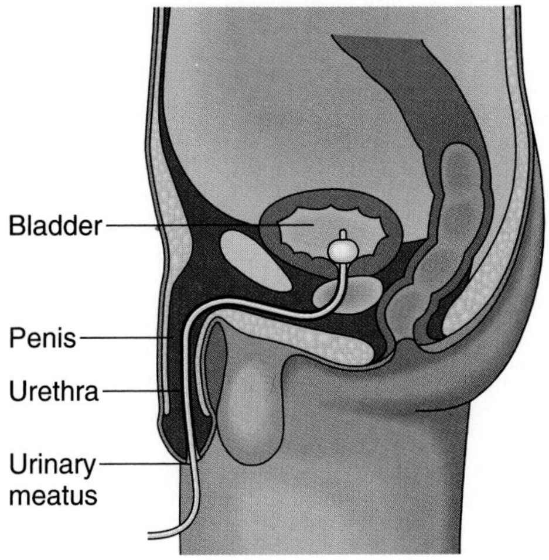

Bladder

Penis

Urethra

Urinary meatus

Figure 3.11 Side view of male anatomy with indwelling urinary catheter in place.

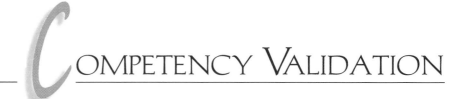

COMPETENCY VALIDATION

Skill: Inserting an Indwelling Urinary Catheter in a Female Patient

Name _____

Preceptor _____

Date _____

Competency Statement   Inserts an indwelling urinary catheter in a female patient while demonstrating correct sterile technique.

Not Competent: _____ 1. Is <u>unable to state reason</u> for task and <u>needs instructions</u> to perform task.

_____ 2. Understands reason for task but <u>needs instructions</u> to perform task.

Competent: _____ 3. Understands reason for task and is able to perform task but <u>needs to increase speed.</u>

_____ 4. Understands reason for task and is able to perform task <u>proficiently.</u>

Performance Criteria

The caregiver demonstrates the ability to do the following:

_____ 1. Wash hands.

_____ 2. Explain the procedure to the patient, emphasizing the need to maintain the sterile field.

_____ 3. Determine if the patient is allergic to iodine-based antiseptics.

_____ 4. Provide for privacy.

_____ 5. Position the patient in the dorsal recumbent position with knees flexed, exposing the labia.

_____ 6. Drape the patient so that only the perineum is exposed.

_____ 7. Remove the full drape from the kit with your fingertips, and place, plastic side down, just under the patient's buttocks (ask her to raise her hips).

_____ 8. Put on sterile gloves.

_____ 9. Prepare the items in the kit for use during insertion, maintaining sterile technique.

_____ 10. Test the balloon for defects. Deflate the balloon, and leave the syringe on the catheter. Liberally lubricate the catheter tip.

_____ 11. With nondominant hand, separate the labia minora, and hold this position until the catheter is inserted. (Note: The dominant hand is the only sterile hand now; the contaminated hand continues to separate the labia.)

_____ 12. Using cotton balls, cleanse the meatus with the aseptic solution:
   a. Making one downward stroke with each cotton ball, begin at the labia on the side farthest from you, and move toward the labia nearest you.
   b. Afterward, wipe once down the center of the meatus.
   c. Wipe once with each cotton ball, and discard.

_____ 13. Insert the tip of the catheter slowly through the urethral opening 3 to 4 inches or until urine returns.

_____ 14. Advance the catheter another .5 to 1.0 inches.

_____ 15. Inflate the balloon with the attached syringe, and gently pull back on the catheter until it stops, or catches.

_____ 16. Measure the amount of urine in the drainage bag, and record.

_____ 17. Remove and discard gloves; wash hands.

_____ 18. Document and report the results to the RN or preceptor.

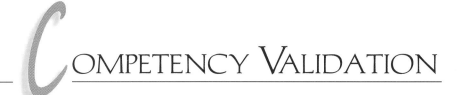

COMPETENCY VALIDATION

Skill: Inserting an Indwelling Urinary Catheter in a Male Patient

Name _____

Preceptor _____

Date _____

Competency Statement   Inserts an indwelling urinary catheter in a male patient while demonstrating correct sterile technique.

Not Competent: _____ 1. Is <u>unable to state reason</u> for task and <u>needs instructions</u> to perform task.

_____ 2. Understands reason for task but <u>needs instructions</u> to perform task.

Competent: _____ 3. Understands reason for task and is able to perform task but <u>needs to increase speed.</u>

_____ 4. Understands reason for task and is able to perform task <u>proficiently.</u>

Performance Criteria

The caregiver demonstrates the ability to do the following:

_____ 1. Wash hands.

_____ 2. Explain the procedure to the patient.

_____ 3. Determine if the patient is allergic to iodine-based antiseptics.

_____ 4. Provide for privacy.

_____ 5. Assemble the equipment, and put on gloves.

_____ 6. Prepare the items in the kit for use during insertion, maintaining sterile technique.

_____ 7. Test the balloon for defects. Deflate the balloon, and leave the syringe attached to the catheter. Liberally lubricate the catheter tip.

_____ 8. Remove the fenestrated drape from the kit, and using nondominant hand, place the penis through the hole in the drape. *Keep dominant hand sterile.*

_____ 9. Pull the penis up at a 90-degree angle to the patient's supine body.

_____ 10. With nondominant hand, gently grasp the glans (tip) of the penis; retract the foreskin if uncircumcised.

_____ 11. Using cotton balls, cleanse the meatus and the glans with aseptic solution, beginning at the urethral opening and moving toward the shaft of the penis; make one complete circle around the penis with each cotton ball. Using the forceps to hold the cotton ball is an optional technique.

_____ 12. Insert the tip of the catheter slowly through the urethral opening to the bifurcation (Y) of the catheter.

_____ 13. Inflate the balloon with the attached syringe, and gently pull back on the catheter until it stops, or catches.

_____ 14. Replace the foreskin of the penis on uncircumcised males.

_____ 15. Measure the amount of urine in the drainage bag, and record.

_____ 16. Remove and discard gloves; wash hands.

_____ 17. Document and report the results to the RN or preceptor.

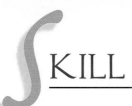

SKILL

Discontinuing an Indwelling Urinary Catheter

Purpose The indwelling urinary catheter is removed when it is determined by the physician or by protocol that the patient is able to urinate on his or her own. It is also removed when the catheter needs to be changed for infection control or due to blockage.

The caregiver demonstrates the ability to do the following:

1. Gather the correct supplies.

2. Communicate using a style that reduces the patient's anxiety.

3. Correctly deflate the retention balloon before removing the catheter.

4. Record the amount of urine left in the drainage bag.

5. Report the results of the procedure to the RN or preceptor.

Drainage Bag The bag that urine from the bladder drains into. It is attached to the indwelling catheter and collects the urine that drains from the bladder.

Retention Balloon The device that holds an indwelling urinary catheter in place in the bladder. It is filled with sterile saline solution. When the saline is removed, that section of the catheter collapses and becomes a narrow tube that can slide through the urethra.

Protective pad or towel • Clean gloves • 10-cc syringe • Washcloth

* Removing an indwelling urinary catheter requires a physician's order in most cases.

* Patients are often happy to have the tube removed but are hesitant that it will hurt. Be honest. Prepare the patient for a stinging sensation and then a feeling of relief when the catheter is out.

* Provide for privacy by closing the door or pulling the curtain.

* Provide for comfort by placing a pad under the patient to catch any urine that may drip during the procedure. Clean the patient's skin if needed.

* Note the condition of the tip of the catheter when you remove it. Be sure it is intact.

* If you note any white to green sediment, notify the RN or physician. This may indicate an infection in progress and may require a culture collection.

When removing a urinary catheter from a child, be honest and explain that the process might sting. Trust is a very important issue for children. If they cannot trust you, they will not feel secure in future interactions. Adolescents, adults, and the elderly may worry that they will not be able to urinate on their own once a catheter is removed. Reassure them that in the majority of cases, this is not a problem.

*C*are must be taken to properly deflate the retention balloon while holding the catheter. A catheter accidentally can be retracted into a male's urethra if the catheter is improperly cut to deflate the balloon. Should this occur, removal from the bladder requires cystoscopic surgery or radiological interventions. Remove the catheter using a slow, steady movement to minimize the patient's pain or discomfort.

1. Wash hands.
2. Explain the procedure to, and provide privacy for, the patient.
3. Gather the supplies.
4. Tuck a protective pad or towel under the patient's hips to catch any urine that may drip during the procedure.
5. Put on gloves.
6. Attach the syringe to the urinary catheter port, and draw back 10 cc of sterile saline solution (Figure 3.12). Be sure to remove all of the solution from the port to allow the balloon to collapse and the catheter to slip easily out of the urethra.
7. Tell the patient that you are ready to gently but firmly pull the catheter out. Encourage the patient to take a deep breath.
8. Clean up any urine that may have dripped.
9. Empty the drainage bag, and record the amount and characteristics of the urine.
10. Discard the catheter and the empty drainage bag in the trash.
11. Remove and discard gloves; wash hands.
12. Document and report the results to the RN or preceptor.

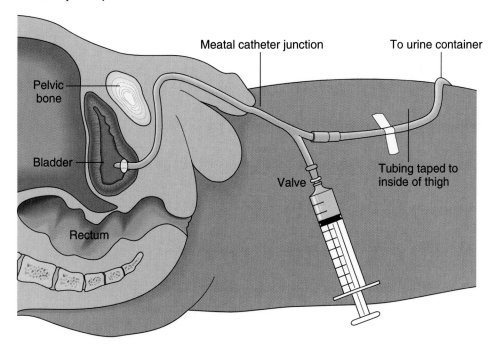

Figure 3.12 Removing an indwelling urinary catheter. Always deflate the retention balloon before removing the catheter.

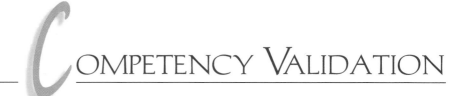

COMPETENCY VALIDATION

Skill: Discontinuing an Indwelling Urinary Catheter

Name _____

Preceptor _____

Date _____

Competency Statement

Discontinues an indwelling urinary catheter while demonstrating correct sterile technique.

Not Competent: _____ 1. Is <u>unable to state reason</u> for task and <u>needs instructions</u> to perform task.

_____ 2. Understands reason for task but <u>needs instructions</u> to perform task.

Competent: _____ 3. Understands reason for task and is able to perform task but <u>needs to increase speed.</u>

_____ 4. Understands reason for task and is able to perform task <u>proficiently.</u>

Performance Criteria

The caregiver demonstrates the ability to do the following:

_____ 1. Wash hands.

_____ 2. Explain the procedure to, and provide privacy for, the patient.

_____ 3. Gather the supplies.

_____ 4. Tuck a protective pad or towel under the patient's hips to catch any urine that may drip during the procedure.

_____ 5. Put on gloves.

_____ 6. Attach the syringe to the urinary catheter port, and draw back 10 cc of sterile saline solution. Be sure to remove all of the solution from the port to allow the balloon to collapse and the catheter to slip easily out of the urethra.

_____ 7. Tell the patient that you are ready to gently but firmly pull the catheter out. Encourage the patient to take a deep breath.

_____ 8. Clean up any urine that may have dripped.

_____ 9. Empty the drainage bag, and record the amount and characteristics of the urine.

_____ 10. Discard the catheter and the empty drainage bag in the trash.

_____ 11. Remove and discard gloves; wash hands.

_____ 12. Document and report the results to the RN or preceptor.

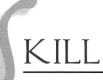

SKILL

Removing Staples

Purpose Staples are commonly used to hold the skin together after a surgical procedure. They allow the edges to come together as the healing process occurs (approximation and granulation). Once the physician has decided that sufficient healing has occurred, the staples are removed. Steri Strips, a type of tape or bandage, are often applied to continue holding the skin together during the later stages of healing to minimize scarring.

The caregiver demonstrates the ability to do the following:

Objectives

1. Gather the correct supplies.

2. Communicate using a style that reduces the patient's anxiety.

3. Maintain sterile technique.

4. Remove staples correctly.

5. Apply Steri Strips correctly.

6. Report the results of the procedure to the RN or preceptor.

Key Terms

Approximation A condition in which the edges of the incision or wound have new growth (granulation) and are sticking together.

Dehiscence A condition in which the edges of the incision, which were to have healed, come apart, revealing underlying levels of skin and tissue.

Evisceration A condition in which the underlying structures below the skin are revealed after dehiscence. Evisceration usually involves the bowel erupting out of the abdominal cavity onto the skin.

Staple A metal device that holds two edges of skin together so that healing can occur.

Staple Extractor A small metal device that slides under the staple in the patient's skin, lifts it up, and pinches it in the middle. Pinching the staple makes the ends rise up out of the skin.

Supplies/ Equipment

Sterile gloves • Steri Strips • Scissors • Skin staple extractor • Skin prep swabs

Pertinent Points

• Removing staples requires a physician's order in most cases.

• Patients are often happy to have the staples removed but are hesitant because they fear that it will hurt. Explain to the patient that there will be a slight, momentary discomfort as the staples are removed but that it usually feels better to have them out.

• Provide for privacy and patient comfort before removing the staples. Close the door or curtain, and check to ensure that the patient is in a comfortable position.

Patients of all ages may be concerned about the appearance of the incision line. Others may focus primarily on getting the staples out. Give the patient time to look at the incision line if desired. Do not say that it looks good or bad, but do say that the wound is healing well if appropriate.

Children may fear mutilation or that the incision will pop open. Adolescents and adults may have body image issues, depending on the location of the incision line. The elderly may fear possible infection and the potential for longer healing times. Diabetic or extremely obese patients are likely to experience more difficulty or slower healing than others.

Key Concept

*W*hen taking the staples out, examine the incision line. If the edges are not approximated and it appears that the incision line is coming undone, **stop** removing the staples and call the nurse or the preceptor to the room immediately with the call bell. Remain with the patient, and stay calm. Dehiscence does not happen often, but always check for it before removing all of the staples.

Steps

1. Wash hands.
2. Explain the procedure to the patient.
3. Provide for privacy.
4. Assemble the equipment (Figure 3.13) and put on gloves.
5. Expose the incision line (remove the old dressing if necessary). Discard the dressing, and change gloves.
6. Open the supplies, and cut the Steri Strips into 2- to 3-inch lengths.
7. Pull on sterile gloves. Remove every other staple. Slide the staple extractor under the staple to lift it, and then squeeze the handles of the extractor to crimp it (Figure 3.14).

Gently lift the staple out of the skin. Note the healing progress.

8. Swab the skin with a prep swab; allow the area to dry thoroughly.
9. Apply a Steri Strip to each place where a staple was removed (Figure 3.15).
10. Remove the remaining staples one at a time.
11. Apply the rest of the Steri Strips to cover the incision line.
12. Remove and discard gloves; wash hands.
13. Document and report the results to the RN or preceptor.

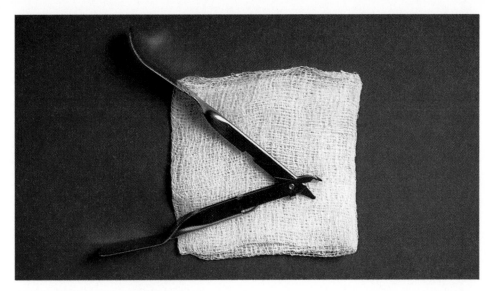

Figure 3.13 Staple removal kit.

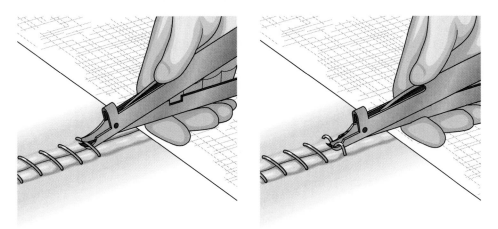

Figure 3.14 Removing staples from an incision line.

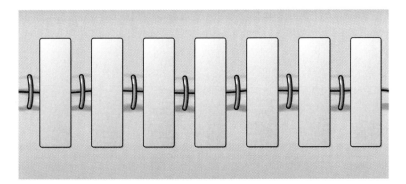

Figure 3.15 Incision line with alternating staples and Steri Strips. Apply a Steri Strip immediately after removing each staple.

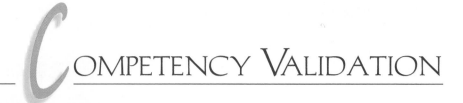

COMPETENCY VALIDATION

Skill: Removing Staples

Name _____

Preceptor _____

Date _____

Competency Statement Removes staples while demonstrating correct sterile technique.

Not Competent: _____ 1. Is <u>unable to state reason</u> for task and <u>needs instructions</u> to perform task.

_____ 2. Understands reason for task but <u>needs instructions</u> to perform task.

Competent: _____ 3. Understands reason for task and is able to perform task but <u>needs to increase speed.</u>

_____ 4. Understands reason for task and is able to perform task <u>proficiently.</u>

Performance Criteria

The caregiver demonstrates the ability to do the following:

_____ 1. Wash hands.

_____ 2. Explain the procedure to the patient.

_____ 3. Provide for privacy.

_____ 4. Assemble the equipment, and put on gloves.

_____ 5. Expose the incision line (remove the old dressing if necessary). Discard the dressing, and change gloves.

_____ 6. Open the supplies, and cut the Steri Strips into 2- to 3-inch lengths.

_____ 7. Put on sterile gloves. Remove every other staple. Slide the staple extractor under the staple to lift it, and then squeeze the handles of the extractor to crimp it. Gently lift the staple out of the skin. Note the healing progress.

_____ 8. Swab the skin with a prep swab; allow the area to dry thoroughly.

_____ 9. Apply a Steri Strip to each place where a staple was removed.

_____ 10. Remove the remaining staples one at a time.

_____ 11. Apply the rest of the Steri Strips to cover the incision line.

_____ 12. Remove and discard gloves; wash hands.

_____ 13. Document and report the results to the RN or preceptor.

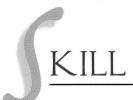

SKILL

Removing Sutures

Purpose Sutures are commonly used to hold the skin together after a surgical procedure or injury to the body. They allow the edges to come together as the healing process occurs (approximation and granulation). Once the physician has decided that sufficient healing has occurred, the sutures are removed. Steri Strips, a type of tape or bandage, are often applied to continue holding the skin together during the later stages of healing to minimize scarring.

The caregiver demonstrates the ability to do the following:

1. Gather the correct supplies.

2. Communicate using a style that reduces the patient's anxiety.

3. Maintain sterile technique.

4. Remove sutures correctly.

5. Apply Steri Strips correctly.

6. Report the results of the procedure to the RN or preceptor.

Objectives

Approximation A condition in which the edges of the incision or wound have new growth (granulation) and are sticking together.

Dehiscence A condition in which the edges of the incision, which were to have healed, come apart, revealing underlying levels of skin and tissue.

Evisceration A condition in which the underlying structures below the skin are revealed after dehiscence. Evisceration usually involves the bowel erupting out of the abdominal cavity onto the skin.

Forceps A metal or plastic device that allows the user to pick up and lift small objects such as sutures.

Sutures A stitch put in place to close a wound or incision.

Key Terms

Sterile gloves • Steri Strips • Scissors • Forceps • Skin prep swabs

Supplies/ Equipment

- Removing sutures requires a physician's order in most cases.

- Patients are often happy to have the sutures removed but are hesitant because they fear that it will hurt. Explain to the patient that there will be a slight, momentary discomfort as the sutures are removed but that it usually feels better to have them out.

- Provide for privacy and patient comfort before removing the sutures. Close the door or curtain, and check to ensure that the patient is in a comfortable position.

Pertinent Points

Age-Specific Considerations

Patients of all ages may be concerned about the appearance of the incision line. Others may focus primarily on getting the sutures out. Give the patient time to look at the incision line if desired. Do not say that it looks good or bad, but do say that the wound is healing well if appropriate.

Children may fear mutilation or that the incision will pop open. Adolescents and adults may have body image issues, depending on the location of the incision line. The elderly may fear possible infection and the potential for longer healing times. Diabetic or extremely obese patients are likely to experience more difficulty or slower healing than others.

Key Concept

*W*hen taking the sutures out, examine the incision line. If the edges are not approximated and it appears that the incision line is coming undone, stop removing the sutures and call the nurse or preceptor to the room immediately with the call bell. Remain with the patient, and stay calm. Dehiscence does not happen often, but always check for it before removing all of the sutures.

Steps

1. Wash hands.
2. Explain the procedure to the patient.
3. Provide for privacy.
4. Assemble the equipment (Figure 3.16), and put on gloves.

5. Expose the suture or the incision line (remove the old dressing if necessary). Discard the dressing, and change gloves.
6. Open the supplies, and cut the Steri Strips into 2- to 3-inch lengths.

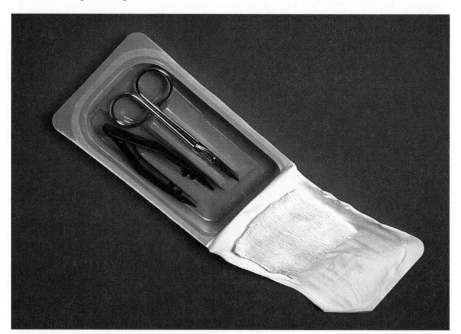

Figure 3.16 Suture removal kit.

7. Put on sterile gloves. Remove every other suture (Figure 3.17). Lift the suture with the forceps, and then cut it with the scissors (Figure 3.18). Be sure to remove both pieces of suture with the forceps by gently lifting them out of the skin. Note the healing progress.

8. Swab the skin with a prep swab; allow the area to dry thoroughly.

9. Apply a Steri Strip to each place where a suture was removed.

10. Remove the remaining sutures one at a time (Figure 3.18).

11. Apply the rest of the Steri Strips to cover the incision line.

12. Remove and discard gloves; wash hands.

13. Document and report the results to the RN or preceptor.

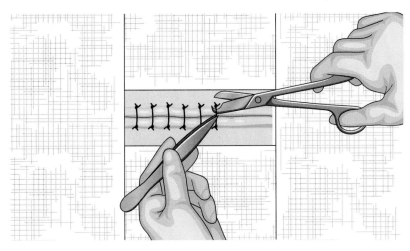

Figure 3.17 Removing sutures from an incision line.

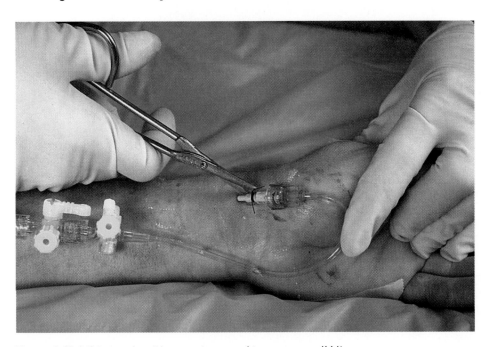

Figure 3.18 Lifting and cutting a suture used to secure an IV line.

COMPETENCY VALIDATION

Skill: Removing Sutures

Name _____

Preceptor _____

Date _____

Competency Statement Removes suture while demonstrating correct sterile technique.

Not Competent: _____ 1. Is <u>unable to state reason</u> for task and <u>needs instructions</u> to perform task.

_____ 2. Understands reason for task but <u>needs instructions</u> to perform task.

Competent: _____ 3. Understands reason for task and is able to perform task but <u>needs to increase speed.</u>

_____ 4. Understands reason for task and is able to perform task <u>proficiently.</u>

Performance Criteria

The caregiver demonstrates the ability to do the following:

_____ 1. Wash hands.

_____ 2. Explain the procedure to the patient.

_____ 3. Provide for privacy.

_____ 4. Assemble the equipment, and put on gloves.

_____ 5. Expose the incision line (remove the old dressing if necessary). Discard the dressing, and change gloves.

_____ 6. Open the supplies, and cut the Steri Strips into 2- to 3-inch lengths.

_____ 7. Put on sterile gloves. Remove every other suture. Lift the suture with the forceps, and then cut it with the scissors. Be sure to remove both pieces of suture with the forceps by gently lifting them out of the skin. Note the healing progress.

_____ 8. Swab the skin with a prep swab; allow the area to dry thoroughly.

_____ 9. Apply a Steri Strip to each place where a suture was removed.

_____ 10. Remove the remaining sutures one at a time.

_____ 11. Apply the rest of the Steri Strips to cover the incision line.

_____ 12. Remove and discard gloves; wash hands.

_____ 13. Document and report the results to the RN or preceptor.

SKILL

Suctioning a Tracheostomy

Purpose Tracheal suctioning is an important procedure that removes thick secretions that have accumulated in a patient's lungs. Because a patient with a tracheostomy has lost the protective filtering function usually performed by the nose, irritants in the air can directly enter the lungs. This often leads to increased secretions, increased mucus, and the formation of crusts. The lungs are challenged to remove these extra particles on their own. Tracheostomy patients may also have underlying medical conditions that increase secretions and mucus or make it difficult for patients to expel them on their own. Failure to remove these irritants can lead to infection, pneumonia, or severe respiratory distress.

Suctioning with a soft rubber catheter assists the tracheostomy patient by removing these secretions, mucus, and small crusts. The caregiver inserts the catheter into the trachea for a short time and then withdraws it. Suctioning removes some secretions from the lungs and stimulates the patient to cough violently. This coughing also helps the patient expel secretions, debris, and mucus.

Because suctioning is a difficult procedure for the patient, it must only be performed when necessary. Indications that a patient may need to be suctioned include an increased rate and frequency of respiration, more difficult, labored respiration, and noisy, gurgling respirations.

The caregiver demonstrates the ability to do the following: Objectives

1. Gather the correct supplies.

2. Communicate using a style that reduces the patient's anxiety.

3. State when to suction a patient.

4. State ways to minimize complications from tracheal suctioning.

5. Competently suction a tracheostomy.

6. Report the results of the procedure to the RN or preceptor.

Hypoxia An inadequate amount of oxygen in the blood.   Key Terms

Tracheostomy A surgical opening in the trachea (windpipe) that leads directly to the lungs, allowing the patient to breathe directly from the lungs.

Wall suction • Goggles • Catheter and glove kit (sterile gloves, sterile small   Supplies/
basin, 14–16F suction catheter) • 500-cc bottle of normal saline (sterile)   Equipment

• Patients consider procedures that interfere with breathing to be very invasive.   Pertinent
  Suctioning is a traumatic experience for the patient because the catheter   Points
  removes air from the lungs as well as any secretions. Help relieve the patient's
  anxiety by describing every step you take.

- Take time and care while performing this procedure. Although suctioning is routine for caregivers, it is not routine for patients.
- Be prepared, and have all of your equipment and supplies ready.
- Maintaining sterile technique is very important. Suctioning introduces a foreign object (the catheter) deep into a body cavity.
- Safe suction pressure for an adult is 80 to 140 mmHg.
- The size of the suction catheter should not be more than one half the diameter of the tracheostomy. Remember, the larger the catheter, the more oxygen will be removed during suctioning.
- As you insert the catheter into the patient's lungs, do not apply any suction. This helps prevent trauma to the mucosal tissue of the lungs.
- Keep the suction catheter in the lungs for no more than 10 to 15 seconds.
- When you withdraw the catheter, twirl it and apply suction intermittently to prevent the catheter from adhering to the tissue.
- Do not introduce the catheter into the patient's lungs more than three times. After this point, the rinse (normal saline) will be fairly contaminated. This precaution helps prevent infection for the patient.

Age-Specific Considerations

Patients of all ages will have concerns about suctioning. Being unable to breathe is a frightening experience. Explain the procedure so that the patient can understand. Show respect and concern for patients by addressing them using the name they have asked you to use.

As people age, the lungs become less elastic, or able to expand. The membranes become thicker, making the exchange of oxygen more difficult. For these reasons, suctioning is a more traumatic process for the elderly. Allow elderly patients more time to catch their breath between insertions of the suction catheter into the tracheostomy.

Key Concepts

- Suctioning is a traumatic procedure for the patient. Only suction when it is necessary.
- Infection and lack of oxygen are two common complications of suctioning that can be minimized.
- The patient cannot breathe while being suctioned. The whole process must last no longer than 10 to 15 seconds. This time limit will help prevent hypoxia, or lack of oxygen, for the patient. Putting the oxygen back on the patient as soon as the suction catheter is out of the tracheostomy will also help prevent hypoxia.
- Hold your breath while you insert the catheter into the tracheostomy. This will give you an indication of how long the patient will be without oxygen during the suctioning process. Remember that patients who are compromised by illness or age usually cannot hold their breath as long as you can.

1. Wash hands, and gather the supplies.

2. Explain the procedure to, and provide privacy for, the patient.

3. Turn on the wall suction. Make sure the pressure is between 80 and 140 mmHg for patient safety.

4. Put on goggles.

5. Loosen the patient's oxygen mask. Leave it in place until ready to suction.

6. Open the catheter kit in a sterile manner. Pour the normal saline into the sterile basin.

7. Put on gloves. Determine which hand will guide the catheter into the tracheostomy; this hand must remain sterile to the patient.

8. Attach the catheter to the suction tubing from the wall suction, holding the tubing with the nonsterile hand and the suction catheter with the sterile hand.

9. Remove the patient's oxygen mask with the nonsterile hand.

10. With the sterile hand, insert the catheter in the airway, without applying suction, until a cough reflex is stimulated or resistance is felt (approximately 6 inches) (Figure 3.19).

11. Withdraw the catheter ½ to 1 inch before applying suction. Withdraw by twisting the catheter with your forefinger and thumb.

12. Apply suction for no more than 10 to 15 seconds.

13. Repeat steps 10 to 12 no more than twice. Allow time between suction episodes for the patient to reoxygenate (apply oxygen mask with nonsterile hand.) Between suction episodes, rinse the end of the catheter in the sterile saline basin. Apply suction to rinse the normal saline through the entire suction catheter tubing.

14. Remove and discard gloves.

15. Document the procedure, and report the color and amount of secretions, as well as how the patient tolerated the procedure, to the RN or preceptor.

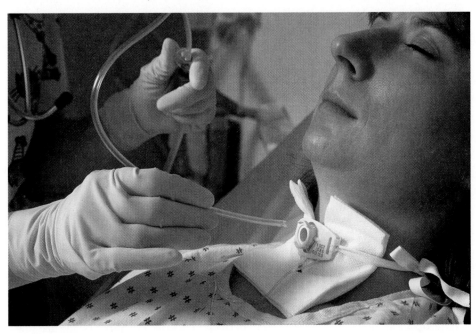

Figure 3.19 Suctioning a tracheostomy.

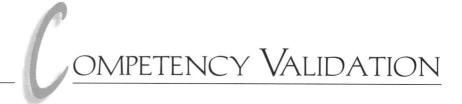

COMPETENCY VALIDATION

Skill: Suctioning a Tracheostomy

Name _____

Preceptor _____

Date _____

Competency Statement

Suctions a tracheostomy while demonstrating correct sterile technique.

Not Competent: _____ 1. Is <u>unable to state reason</u> for task and <u>needs instructions</u> to perform task.

_____ 2. Understands reason for task but <u>needs instructions</u> to perform task.

Competent: _____ 3. Understands reason for task and is able to perform task but <u>needs to increase speed.</u>

_____ 4. Understands reason for task and is able to perform task <u>proficiently.</u>

Performance Criteria

The caregiver demonstrates the ability to do the following:

_____ 1. Wash hands, and gather the supplies.

_____ 2. Explain the procedure to the patient.

_____ 3. Turn on the wall suction. Make sure the pressure is between 80 and 140 mmHg for patient safety.

_____ 4. Put on goggles.

_____ 5. Loosen the patient's oxygen mask. Leave it in place until ready to suction.

_____ 6. Open the catheter kit in a sterile manner. Pour the normal saline into the sterile basin.

_____ 7. Put on gloves. Determine which hand will guide the catheter into the tracheostomy; this hand must remain sterile to the patient.

_____ 8. Attach the catheter to the suction tubing from the wall suction, holding the tubing with the non-sterile hand and the suction catheter with the sterile hand.

_____ 9. Remove the patient's oxygen mask with the nonsterile hand.

_____ 10. With the sterile hand, insert the catheter in the airway, without applying suction, until a cough reflex is stimulated or resistance is felt (approximately 6 inches).

_____ 11. Withdraw the catheter ½ to 1 inch, twisting the catheter with your forefinger and thumb.

_____ 12. Apply suction for no more than 10 to 15 seconds.

_____ 13. Repeat steps 10 to 12 no more than twice. Allow time between suction episodes for the patient to reoxygenate. (Apply oxygen mask with nonsterile hand.) Between suction episodes, rinse the end of the catheter in the sterile saline basin. Apply suction to rinse the normal saline through the entire suction catheter tubing.

_____ 14. Remove and discard gloves.

_____ 15. Document the procedure, and report the color and amount of secretions, as well as how the patient tolerated the procedure, to the RN or preceptor.

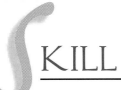

SKILL

Performing Tracheostomy Care

Purpose   Tracheostomy care is given to prevent a buildup of secretions and crustations from forming on the trach. This helps prevent infection and clogging of the trach. A clogged trach will prevent the patient from breathing. There are two types of trach care. One type is used when the patient has a nondisposable (metal or plastic) inner cannula (Figure 3.20) and the other is used when the patient has a disposable (plastic) inner cannula (Figure 3.21).

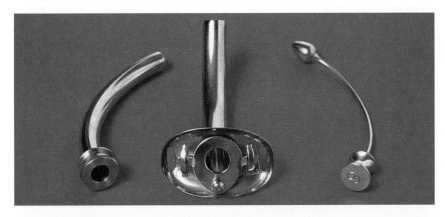

Figure 3.20 Nondisposable trach.

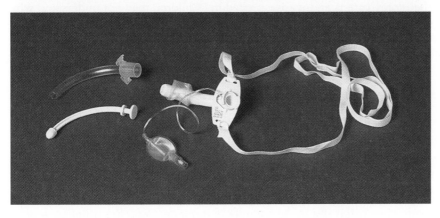

Figure 3.21 Disposable trach.

The caregiver demonstrates the ability to do the following:

1. Gather the correct supplies.

2. Communicate using a style that reduces the patient's anxiety.

3. State when to perform trach care.

4. Maintain sterile technique.

5. Perform the procedure correctly.

6. Report the results of the procedure to the RN or preceptor.

Disposable Inner Cannula The inner tube of the trach set that is thrown away and replaced with a clean one during trach care.

Key Terms

Flange The metal plate section of the trach that holds the trach set flush to the skin. The trach ties attach to the flange.

Nondisposable Inner Cannula The inner tube of the trach set that is cleaned and replaced using sterile technique when performing trach care.

Obturator The wire or plastic guide that is used when first inserting the trach set.

Outer Cannula The larger tube of the trach set that stays in the patient.

Nondisposable Inner Cannula

Trach care kit • Peroxide and saline solutions (sterile) • Sterile gloves • 4-by-4-inch gauze • Sterile cotton-tip applicators • Trach pants (drain sponge)

Disposable Inner Cannula

Trach care kit, with a replacement inner cannula • Peroxide and saline solutions (sterile) • Sterile gloves • Sterile cotton-tip applicators • Trach pants (drain sponge) • 4-by-4-inch gauze

- Trach care is a very important procedure for keeping the patient's airway clean and protecting against infection.
- Sterile technique must be maintained throughout the procedure.
- Because the patient's oxygen will not be on during the procedure, speed is important.

Patients of all ages will have concerns about tracheostomy care. Explain the procedure so that the patient can understand. Show respect and concern for patients by addressing them using the name they have asked you to use. Take time and care while performing the procedure. Although trach care is routine for caregivers, it is not routine for patients or their families.

Tracheostomy care is an invasive procedure. Children may not understand why it is necessary or what is happening when caregivers perform the procedure. Adolescents, adults, and the elderly will understand the need for cleanliness but may still fear the procedure. Be understanding of the feelings of your patients.

Some patients need extra oxygen to assist with breathing, and many also need it to help humidify the air, a function that is lost when the air is not filtered and warmed by the nose. Both functions are compromised during trach care. If at any time the patient's respiratory status is compromised, check that the inner cannula is in place. Stop the process, and call for assistance.

Steps for
Performing
Tracheostomy
Care with a
Nondisposable
Inner Cannula

1. Wash hands.
2. Explain the procedure to the patient.
3. Provide for privacy.
4. Assemble the equipment (Figure 3.22). Open the trach care kit, and prepare the sterile field. Organize your supplies and equipment.
5. Pour the peroxide solution into one container, and the saline solution into the other.
6. Put on gloves.
7. Hold the flange with one hand, and unlock the inner cannula by twisting it to the open position. Carefully withdraw the inner cannula with an

upward arc without touching the inside of the cannula.

8. Inspect the inner cannula for crustations and mucus, then put it in the peroxide solution.

9. Use the wire brush to clean the inner cannula, then put the cannula in the saline solution to rinse. Dry it thoroughly with the gauze (Figure 3.23a).

10. Holding the outer rim, gently reinsert the cannula, and twist it to lock it into place (Figure 3.23b).

11. Clean the flange with the peroxide and rinse it with the saline solution, using the cotton-tip applicators. Apply the trach pants (drain sponge) around the flange (Figure 3.23c).

12. Dispose of the supplies. Remove and discard gloves; wash hands.

13. Document and report the results to the RN or preceptor.

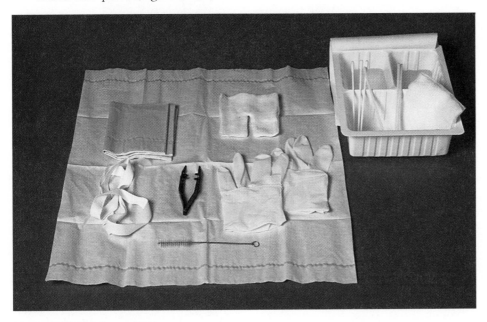

Figure 3.22 Trach care kit.

1. Wash hands.

2. Explain the procedure to the patient.

3. Provide for privacy.

4. Assemble the equipment (Figure 3.22). Open the trach care kit, and prepare the sterile field.

5. Pour the peroxide solution into one container, and the saline solution into the other.

6. Put on gloves.

7. Hold the flange with one hand, and unlock or pinch open the inner cannula. Carefully withdraw the inner cannula with an upward arc.

8. Inspect the inner cannula for crustations and mucus, then dispose of it.

9. Insert the new inner cannula by grasping the outer rim and inserting gently. Clip the inner cannula onto the rim.

10. Clean the flange with peroxide and rinse it with the saline solution, using the cotton-tip applicators.

11. Dispose of the supplies. Remove and discard gloves; wash hands.

12. Document and report the results to the RN or preceptor.

Steps for Performing Tracheostomy Care with a Disposable Inner Cannula

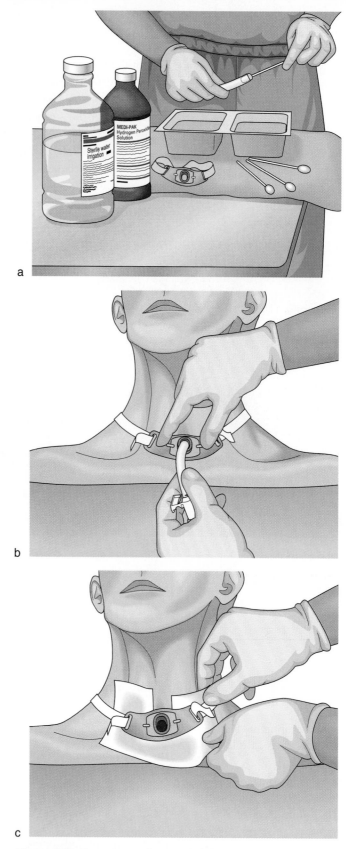

Figure 3.23 Steps in trach care: (a) cleaning the inner cannula, (b) reinserting the inner cannula, (c) replacing the trach pants.

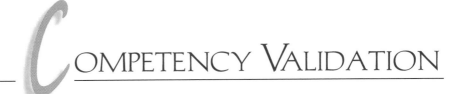

COMPETENCY VALIDATION

Skill: Performing Tracheostomy Care with a Nondisposable Inner Cannula

Name _____

Preceptor _____

Date _____

Competency Statement Performs tracheostomy care with a nondisposable inner cannula while demonstrating correct sterile technique.

Not Competent: _____ 1. Is <u>unable to state reason</u> for task and <u>needs instructions</u> to perform task.

_____ 2. Understands reason for task but <u>needs instructions</u> to perform task.

Competent: _____ 3. Understands reason for task and is able to perform task but <u>needs to increase speed.</u>

_____ 4. Understands reason for task and is able to perform task <u>proficiently.</u>

Performance Criteria

The caregiver demonstrates the ability to do the following:

_____ 1. Wash hands.

_____ 2. Explain the procedure to the patient.

_____ 3. Provide for privacy.

_____ 4. Assemble the equipment. Open the trach care kit, and prepare the sterile field. Organize your supplies and equipment.

_____ 5. Pour the peroxide solution into one container, and the saline solution into the other.

_____ 6. Put on gloves.

_____ 7. Hold the flange with one hand, and unlock the inner cannula by twisting it to the open position. Carefully withdraw the inner cannula with an upward arc without touching the inside of the cannula.

_____ 8. Inspect the inner cannula for crustations and mucus, then put it in the peroxide solution.

_____ 9. Use the wire brush to clean the inner cannula, then put the cannula in the saline solution to rinse. Dry it thoroughly with the gauze.

_____ 10. Holding the outer rim, gently reinsert the cannula, and twist it to lock it into place.

_____ 11. Clean the flange with the peroxide and rinse it with the saline solution, using the cotton-tip applicators. Apply the trach pants (drain sponge) around the flange.

_____ 12. Dispose of the supplies. Remove and discard gloves; wash hands.

_____ 13. Document and report the results to the RN or preceptor.

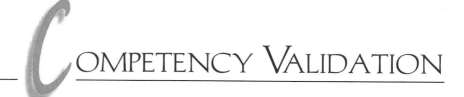

COMPETENCY VALIDATION

Skill: Performing Tracheostomy Care with a Disposable Inner Cannula

Name _____

Preceptor _____

Date _____

Competency Statement

Performs tracheostomy care with a disposable inner cannula while demonstrating correct sterile technique.

Not Competent: _____ 1. Is <u>unable to state reason</u> for task and <u>needs instructions</u> to perform task.

_____ 2. Understands reason for task but <u>needs instructions</u> to perform task.

Competent: _____ 3. Understands reason for task and is able to perform task but <u>needs to increase speed.</u>

_____ 4. Understands reason for task and is able to perform task <u>proficiently.</u>

Performance Criteria

The caregiver demonstrates the ability to do the following:

_____ 1. Wash hands.

_____ 2. Explain the procedure to the patient.

_____ 3. Provide for privacy.

_____ 4. Assemble the equipment. Open the trach care kit, and prepare the sterile field.

_____ 5. Pour the peroxide solution into one container, and the saline solution into the other.

_____ 6. Put on gloves.

_____ 7. Hold the flange with one hand, and unlock or pinch open the inner cannula. Carefully withdraw the inner cannula with an upward arc.

_____ 8. Inspect the inner cannula for crustations and mucus, then dispose of it.

_____ 9. Insert the new inner cannula by grasping the outer rim and inserting gently. Clip the inner cannula onto the rim.

_____ 10. Clean the flange with peroxide and rinse it with saline solution, using the cotton-tip applicators.

_____ 11. Dispose of the supplies. Remove and discard gloves; wash hands.

_____ 12. Document and report the results to the RN or preceptor.

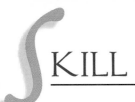

SKILL

Performing Tracheostomy Stoma Care

Purpose Patients who have tracheostomies often experience a buildup of secretions or crusts around their stoma. Built-up secretions can interfere with the patient's ability to breathe. This may occur with either a disposable or a nondisposable trach (see Figures 3.20 and 3.21). Stoma care is the process to remove these secretions, crusts, or other debris from under the flange of the trach and from around the stoma.

The caregiver demonstrates ability to do the following:

Objectives

1. Gather the correct supplies.

2. Communicate using a style that reduces the patient's anxiety.

3. State when to perform stoma care.

4. Maintain sterile technique.

5. Perform the procedure correctly.

6. Report the results of the procedure to the RN or preceptor.

Stoma A surgically created opening to the trachea that serves as an airway.

Key Term

Peroxide and saline solutions • 2 small sterile containers • Sterile cotton-tip applicators • Trach pants (drain sponge)

Supplies/ Equipment

- Trach care is a very important procedure for keeping the patient's airway clean and protecting against infection.

- Sterile technique must be maintained throughout the procedure.

- If at any time the patient's respiratory status is compromised, check that the inner cannula is in place. Stop the procedure, and call for assistance.

Pertinent Points

Patients of all ages will have concerns about tracheostomy stoma care. Explain the procedure so that the patient can understand. Show respect and concern for patients by addressing them using the name they have asked you to use. Take time and care while performing the procedure. Although stoma care is routine for caregivers, it is not routine for patients or their families.

Age-Specific Considerations

Tracheostomy stoma care is a potentially irritating procedure. Children may not understand why it is necessary or what is happening when caregivers begin to clean the area. Adolescents, adults, and the elderly will understand the need for cleanliness but may still fear the procedure.

Key Concept

*I*n most people, the nose serves as a filter during the breathing process. In tracheostomy patients, the stoma provides direct access to the bronchi and the lungs. Therefore, accidentally pushing secretions or crustations into the trach tube when swabbing around the stoma may cause obstruction of the airway or breathing difficulties.

1. Wash hands.
2. Explain the procedure to the patient.
3. Provide for privacy.
4. Assemble the equipment.
5. Pour the peroxide solution into one container, and the saline into the other.
6. Put on gloves.
7. Remove the old, soiled trach pants.
8. Note the condition of the skin and stoma (Figure 3.24). Report any unusual findings to the nurse or preceptor.
9. Apply sterile gloves.
10. Clean the stoma with sterile cotton applicators dipped in peroxide, and then rinse with sterile cotton applicators dipped in saline solution. Rinse the skin thoroughly to prevent irritation. Use each applicator only once. Use a rolling motion to apply the peroxide and to rinse with the saline.
11. Apply the sterile trach pants (Figure 3.23c).
12. Remove and discard gloves; wash hands.
13. Document and report the results to the RN or preceptor.

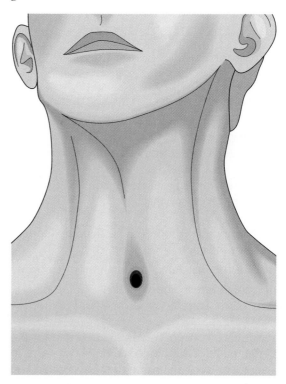

Figure 3.24 Patient with a tracheostomy stoma.

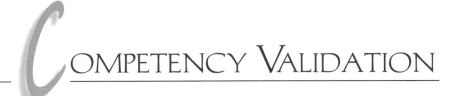

COMPETENCY VALIDATION

Name _____

Preceptor _____

Date _____

Competency Statement   Performs tracheostomy stoma care while demonstrating correct sterile technique.

Not Competent: _____ 1. Is <u>unable to state reason</u> for task and <u>needs instructions</u> to perform task.

_____ 2. Understands reason for task but <u>needs instructions</u> to perform task.

Competent: _____ 3. Understands reason for task and is able to perform task but <u>needs to increase speed.</u>

_____ 4. Understands reason for task and is able to perform task <u>proficiently.</u>

Performance Criteria

The caregiver demonstrates the ability to do the following:

_____ 1. Wash hands.

_____ 2. Explain the procedure to the patient.

_____ 3. Provide for privacy.

_____ 4. Assemble the equipment.

_____ 5. Pour the peroxide solution into one container, and the saline into the other.

_____ 6. Put on gloves.

_____ 7. Remove the old, soiled trach pants.

_____ 8. Note the condition of the skin and stoma. Report any unusual findings to the nurse or preceptor.

_____ 9. Put on sterile gloves.

_____ 10. Clean the stoma with sterile cotton applicators dipped in peroxide, and then rinse with sterile cotton applicators dipped in saline solution. Rinse the skin thoroughly to prevent irritation. Use each applicator only once. Use a rolling motion to apply the peroxide and to rinse with the saline.

_____ 11. Apply the sterile trach pants.

_____ 12. Remove and discard gloves; wash hands.

_____ 13. Document and report the results to the RN or preceptor.

Priming Blood Tubing and Checking Blood Products

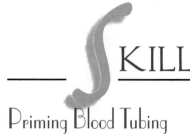

SKILL

Priming Blood Tubing

Purpose Priming the blood tubing before a blood transfusion prevents air from entering the patient's bloodstream. Air of sufficient quantity may result in a serious complication for the patient called *pulmonary embolism*. This condition occurs when the air travels into the pulmonary artery and prevents the artery from receiving oxygen. As a result, the patient becomes short of breath and anxious and may have a cardiac arrest. Priming the tubing involves attaching normal saline solution to one end of the tubing and allowing gravity to push the fluid through the tubing.

Objectives

The caregiver demonstrates the ability to do the following:

1. Gather the correct supplies.

2. Communicate using a style that reduces the patient's anxiety.

3. Maintain sterile technique.

4. Correctly spike the normal saline and flush the tubing.

5. Correctly connect the tubing to the existing IV access site.

6. Report the results of the procedure to the RN or preceptor.

Key Terms

Clamp/Regulator A device on the blood tubing that allows the caregiver to control the speed at which the blood drips into the patient.

Filter A piece of equipment in the blood tubing that keeps the blood product from clumping together as it enters the patient's body.

Port A plastic device on the end of the blood bag that connects it with the end of the blood tubing.

Normal Saline A fluid prepared in a sterile manner that is chemically similar to the fluid in the blood. It allows for the safe transfusion of blood products.

Spike The pointed plastic end of the blood tubing that connects to the port of the blood bag. Pushing the spike into the port is called *spiking*.

Supplies/
Equipment

Blood tubing • Normal saline • IV pole • Clean gloves • Tape

Pertinent
Points

• Explain the procedure to the patient, and answer any questions.

• Ensure the patient's comfort. Ask if the patient needs to use the rest room before beginning the procedure; priming the tubing and the subsequent initiation of the transfusion will be a busy time.

Age-Specific
Considerations

Patients of all ages, particularly children, may fear that the procedure will hurt. Answer any questions, and explain the procedure to the patient.

*C*orrectly identify the patient who is to receive blood, and who is to have the blood tubing prepared by the caregiver.

1. Wash hands.

2. Explain the procedure to the patient.

3. Provide for privacy.

4. Assemble the equipment.

5. Prepare the blood tubing by opening the package and closing the clamp/regulator.

6. Open the bag containing the normal saline, and check the label to be sure it says "Normal Saline."

7. Open the tab on the port of the normal saline, and remove the white cap on the end of the spike of the blood tubing. Connect the port of the normal saline to the spike of the blood tubing. Push and turn to get a tight connection.

8. Hang the normal saline bag on the IV pole (Figure 3.25).

9. Release the clamp/regulator to allow the fluid to flow through the tubing.

10. Close the clamp when the fluid drips out the end of the tubing.

11. Inspect the tubing for air bubbles. If present, open the clamp and let more fluid flush through until the air is pushed out of the tubing.

12. Squeeze the filter to make sure that the level of the fluid is over the top of the filter prongs. Leave adequate room for the blood to drip.

13. Put on gloves, and remove the existing IV dressing. Disconnect the blood tubing at the hub, and connect the other end of the tubing to the IV hub (remove the cap on the end before connecting). Tape the new clean dressing to maintain the IV site.

14. Remove and discard gloves; wash hands.

15. Document and report the results to the RN or preceptor.

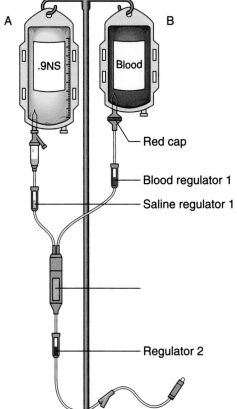

A   .9NS

B   Blood

— Red cap

— Blood regulator 1

— Saline regulator 1

— Regulator 2

Figure 3.25 IV tubing used in blood transfusions has two solution-connection ports—one for the IV solution and one for the blood.

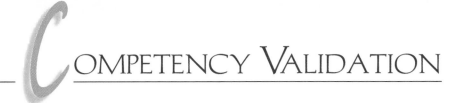

COMPETENCY VALIDATION

Skill: Priming Blood Tubing

Name _____

Preceptor _____

Date _____

Competency Statement   Primes blood tubing while demonstrating correct sterile technique.

Not Competent: _____ 1. Is <u>unable to state reason</u> for task and <u>needs instructions</u> to perform task.

_____ 2. Understands reason for task but <u>needs instructions</u> to perform task.

Competent: _____ 3. Understands reason for task and is able to perform task but <u>needs to increase speed.</u>

_____ 4. Understands reason for task and is able to perform task <u>proficiently.</u>

Performance Criteria

The caregiver demonstrates the ability to do the following:

_____ 1. Wash hands.

_____ 2. Explain the procedure to the patient.

_____ 3. Provide for privacy.

_____ 4. Assemble the equipment.

_____ 5. Prepare the blood tubing by opening the package and closing the clamp/regulator.

_____ 6. Open the bag containing the normal saline, and check the label to be sure it says "Normal Saline."

_____ 7. Open the tab on the port of the normal saline, and remove the white cap on the end of the spike of the blood tubing. Connect the port of the normal saline to the spike of the blood tubing. Push and turn to get a tight connection.

_____ 8. Hang the normal saline bag on the IV pole.

_____ 9. Release the clamp/regulator to allow the fluid to flow through the tubing.

_____ 10. Close the clamp when the fluid drips out the end of the tubing.

_____ 11. Inspect the tubing for air bubbles. If present, open the clamp and let more fluid flush through until the air is pushed out of the tubing.

_____ 12. Squeeze the filter to make sure that the level of the fluid is over the top of the filter prongs. Leave adequate room for the blood to drip.

_____ 13. Put on gloves, and remove the existing IV dressing. Disconnect the blood tubing at the hub, and connect the other end of the tubing to the IV hub (remove the cap on the end before connecting). Tape the new clean dressing to maintain the IV site.

_____ 14. Remove and discard gloves; wash hands.

_____ 15. Document and report the results to the RN or preceptor.

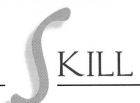

SKILL

Checking Blood Products

Purpose   Errors in matching the right blood to the right patient **can result in death.** Any blood given to a patient must be complementary and safe for the patient to receive. The collection, cross-matching, and typing process that blood administration requires is long and complex. Every effort is made to ensure that the information related to the blood that is collected remains with that unit of blood.

The caregiver demonstrates the ability to do the following:

Objectives

1. Identify the correct patient.

2. Verify the blood product to be administered to the patient.

3. Accurately complete the blood transfusion slip.

Key Terms

Blood Bank Identification Number   The number assigned to the blood product to use in matching it to the patient. The blood bank identification number helps prevent patients from receiving the wrong blood product, which could result in death for the patient.

Blood Slip   A slip of paper that indicates the type of blood product, the patient's blood type, and the expiration date for the product. The blood slip is used to match the patient with the correct blood product.

Blood Type   A unique characteristic of blood. Patients can have A, B, O, or AB type blood. Another characteristic is positive (+) or negative (−) factors. This represents the presence or absence of antigens in the blood.

Expiration Date   The date after which a blood product is no longer safe to give.

Patient Identification Number   The number assigned to the patient by the health care institution. This number is used on all paperwork or records associated with the patient. This process prevents patient records from being mixed up.

Patient name band • Blood slip • Blood product

Supplies/
Equipment

Pertinent
Points

- Patients can only receive like type blood or blood with fewer antigens than they possess. For example, a patient with AB+ blood can receive O− blood. O− blood is considered to be the universal donor and AB+ blood is the most restrictive donor. In most cases, patients receive identically matching blood products to reduce the chance of error and potentially fatal complications for the patient. If you have any questions about whether the blood product is appropriate for a particular patient, contact the blood bank.

- Always check to make sure that the expiration dates on the blood slip and the unit of blood match. Also check to make sure that the blood product has not expired.

- Before beginning the procedure, determine which role you will play: checking the blood product or checking the blood slip. Both associates check the identity of the patient.

- Double-checking the blood assures both the caregivers and the patient that safety precautions are being followed. Explain to the patient that errors are very rare, and that the purpose of the procedure is to ensure safety.

- Use this time to educate the patient about the transfusion procedure used in your institution. Answer any questions that the patient and the family have.

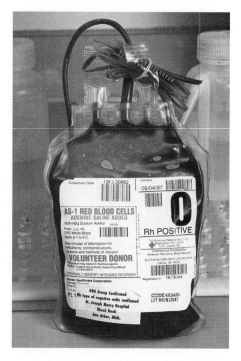

Age-Specific Considerations

Patients of all ages may have concerns, fears, and misconceptions about receiving blood. Address all issues with respect. Explain how the blood can help them, where it came from, and what they can expect to feel. Children as well as adults may fear that the transfusion will hurt.

Key Concepts

- The blood slip contains all of the information regarding the characteristics of the blood and the type of blood that the patient needs. Double-checking the identification of the unit of blood, the patient, and the blood slip reduces the risk that the transfusion will harm the patient.

- It is important to relax and think clearly while checking blood products. If you rush through the procedure, you will not catch errors. Correctly identifying the patient who is to receive blood is crucial for patient safety.

Steps

1. Ask the patient to spell his or her name as you check the spelling on the blood slip and on the patient's name band. (If the patient is unable to spell the name, ask another caregiver to read it aloud from the patient's ID band.)

2. Read aloud the patient identification number on the blood slip as a second caregiver checks it against the ID number on the patient's name band.

3. Read aloud the blood bank identification number, blood type, and expiration date from the blood slip as the second caregiver checks this information against the blood bag (Figure 3.26). Verify blood bank identification number, blood type, and expiration date as second caregiver reads aloud this information from the blood bag.

4. Immediately inform the second caregiver of any discrepancy in the information.

5. Sign you name on the slip, indicating the double-check procedure, and give it to the second caregiver to sign.

Figure 3.26 Blood bag.

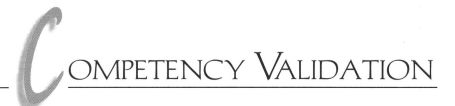

COMPETENCY VALIDATION

Skill: Checking Blood Products

Name _____

Preceptor _____

Date _____

Competency Statement   Checks blood products while demonstrating correct technique.

Not Competent: _____ 1. Is <u>unable to state reason</u> for task and <u>needs instructions</u> to perform task.

_____ 2. Understands reason for task but <u>needs instructions</u> to perform task.

Competent: _____ 3. Understands reason for task and is able to perform task but <u>needs to increase speed.</u>

_____ 4. Understands reason for task and is able to perform task <u>proficiently.</u>

Performance Criteria

The caregiver demonstrates the ability to do the following:

_____ 1. Ask the patient to spell his or her name as you check the spelling on the blood slip and on the patient's name band. (If the patient is unable to spell the name, ask another caregiver to read it aloud from the patient's ID band.)

_____ 2. Read aloud the patient identification number on the blood slip as a second caregiver checks it against the ID number on the patient's name band.

_____ 3. Read aloud the blood bank identification number, blood type, and expiration date from the blood slip as the second caregiver checks this information against the blood bag.

_____ 4. Verify blood bank identification number, blood type, and expiration date as second caregiver reads aloud this information from the blood bag.

_____ 5. Immediately inform the second caregiver of any discrepancy in the information.

_____ 6. Initial the blood slip, indicating the double-check procedure, and give it to the second caregiver to sign.

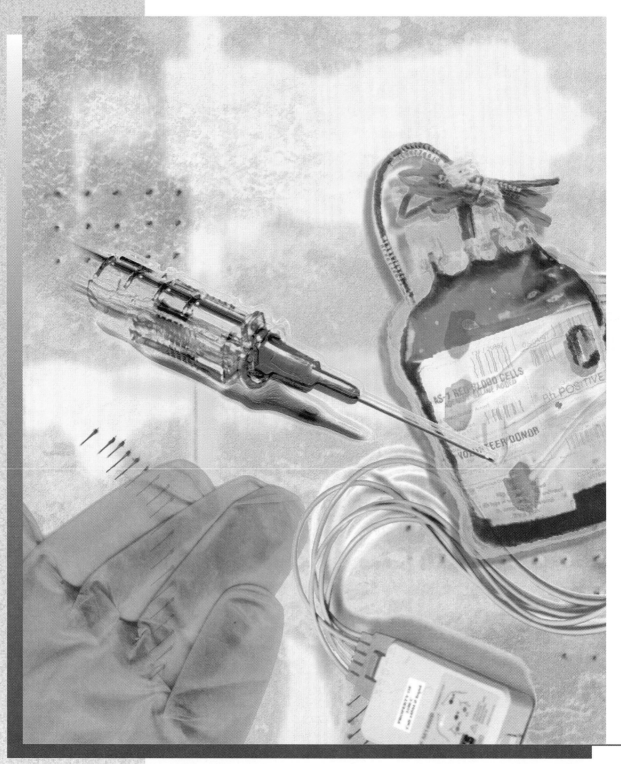

CHAPTER 4
SPECIMEN COLLECTION

Specimen collection is an important component of the caregiver's job. Patients receive treatment and are prescribed medications based on the findings of lab results. Specimens that are collected improperly or are contaminated in the process must frequently be obtained and analyzed again, resulting in unnecessary expense. Therefore, it is always important to acquire the desired specimen, record the correct information on the lab slip, and accurately document the results. The use of standard precautions will prevent unnecessary risk and personal exposure of the caregiver involved in specimen collection or processing.

This chapter prepares caregivers to perform the following skills:

Collecting a Sterile Urine Specimen

Obtaining a Sputum Specimen

Obtaining a Gastric Specimen

Collecting Stool for Hemoccult Testing

Checking Blood Glucose

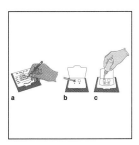
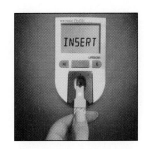
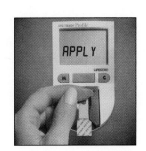

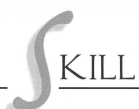

SKILL

Collecting a Sterile Urine Specimen

Purpose   A sterile urine specimen is needed to diagnose and treat many different diseases and disorders. The specimen must be sterile, or free of germs that are on the outside of the body, in order to get an accurate result. The specimen is obtained either by performing the straight catheterization procedure or by clamping an indwelling urinary catheter and withdrawing a sample of urine with a syringe from the tubing.

Objectives

The caregiver demonstrates the ability to do the following:

1. Gather the correct supplies.

2. Communicate using a style that reduces the patient's anxiety.

3. Obtain a sterile urine specimen.

4. Apply the correct lab label.

5. Report the results of the procedure to the RN or preceptor.

Key Term

Specimen Identification The process of ensuring that the correct patient's name is attached to each specimen. This includes identifying the correct patient from whom to obtain the specimen. If the specimen is obtained from the wrong patient, the result could be an inaccurate diagnosis or improper treatment.

Supplies/ Equipment

Gloves • Clamp • Alcohol swabs • 10-cc syringe • Sterile specimen cup • Lab label

Pertinent Points

• Explain to the patient why the specimen is needed and how you will obtain it.

• When using the straight catheterization method, collect the urine in the sterile specimen cup as part of the procedure.

• When clamping an indwelling urinary catheter to collect a urine specimen, note the time the tubing is clamped. Remember to remove the clamp within 15 minutes.

Age-Specific Considerations

Provide privacy, and avoid exposing the patient's genitals while collecting the sterile urine specimen. Ask visitors to step outside the room if that is the patient's preference.

Reassure all patients that collecting the specimen will not cause pain. A child who sees the needle may be fearful and require extra reassurance.

Key Concept

*A*n indwelling urinary catheter that is left clamped may cause pain, infection, or injury to the patient.

1. Wash hands.
2. Identify the correct patient.
3. Explain the procedure to the patient.
4. Assemble the equipment, and put on gloves.
5. Clamp the indwelling urinary catheter below the port by folding the plastic tubing in half and applying a metal or plastic clamp (Figure 4.1).
6. Wait no more than 15 minutes for a small amount of urine to collect in the tubing above the port.
7. Insert a sterile syringe gently into the port (after swabbing it with alcohol), taking care not to poke the needle through the tubing.
8. Withdraw approximately 10 cc of urine (Figure 4.2).
9. Empty the urine from the syringe into the *sterile* specimen cup. Take care not to touch the rim or inside cover of the cap (this prevents contamination of the specimen).
10. Unclamp the catheter tubing, and straighten it out. Be sure that the urine is now freely flowing.
11. Apply the correct lab label to the specimen cup and bag, according to institution policy.
12. Document and report the results to the RN or preceptor.

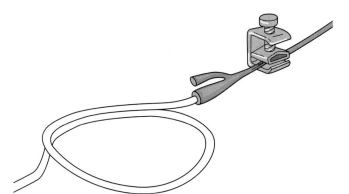

Figure 4.1 Collecting a sterile urine specimen: clamping the catheter tubing.

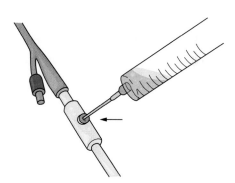

Figure 4.2 Collecting a sterile urine specimen: withdrawing the urine.

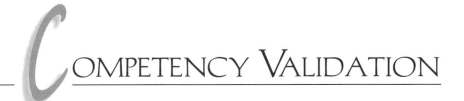

COMPETENCY VALIDATION

Skill: Collecting a Sterile Urine Specimen

Name _____

Preceptor _____

Date _____

Competency Statement

Demonstrates collecting a sterile urine specimen while using correct sterile technique.

Not Competent: _____ 1. Is <u>unable to state reason</u> for task and <u>needs instructions</u> to perform task.

_____ 2. Understands reason for task but <u>needs instructions</u> to perform task.

Competent: _____ 3. Understands reason for task and is able to perform task but <u>needs to increase speed.</u>

_____ 4. Understands reason for task and is able to perform task <u>proficiently.</u>

Performance Criteria

The caregiver demonstrates the ability to do the following:

_____ 1. Wash hands.

_____ 2. Identify the correct patient.

_____ 3. Explain the procedure to the patient.

_____ 4. Assemble the equipment, and apply gloves.

_____ 5. Clamp the indwelling urinary catheter below the port by folding the plastic tubing in half and applying a metal or plastic clamp.

_____ 6. Wait no more than 15 minutes for a small amount of urine to collect in the tubing above the port.

_____ 7. Insert a sterile syringe gently into the port (after swabbing it with alcohol), taking care not to poke the needle through the tubing.

_____ 8. Withdraw approximately 10 cc of urine.

_____ 9. Empty the urine from the syringe into the specimen cup. Take care not to touch the rim or inside cover of the cap (this prevents contamination of the specimen).

_____ 10. Unclamp the tubing, and straighten it out. Be sure that the urine is now freely flowing.

_____ 11. Apply the correct lab label to the specimen cup and bag, according to institution policy.

_____ 12. Document and report the results to the RN or preceptor.

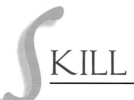

SKILL

Obtaining a Sputum Specimen

Purpose The amount, color, and constituents of the sputum are important in the diagnosis of respiratory illnesses or infections. Sputum specimens are obtained from patients to determine if they have respiratory infections or illnesses, including cancer of the lung, tuberculosis, or pneumonia. The best time to collect a sputum specimen is in the morning. After sleeping, the patient can often more easily expectorate accumulated secretions from the lungs and bronchial tubes.

The caregiver demonstrates the ability to do the following:

1. Gather the correct supplies.

2. Communicate using a style that reduces the patient's anxiety.

3. Obtain a sputum specimen.

4. Apply the correct lab label.

5. Report the results of the procedure to the RN or preceptor.

Expectorate To cough up sputum from the lungs and spit it out of the mouth.

Sputum Secretions or materials coughed up from a patient's lungs. Sputum is thicker than saliva, the moist substance from the patient's mouth, and may contain mucus, pus, blood, or microorganisms.

Gloves • Sputum cup • Tissues • Lab label

- If the patient has eaten recently, it is a good idea to have her rinse her mouth before collecting the specimen. This will prevent food from mixing with the specimen when the patient spits out sputum.
- Have the patient take three or four deep breaths before expectorating. This will help ensure a good sample.

Older adults or young children may need extra assistance providing the sputum specimen. A demonstration of how to take deep breaths and cough up the sputum may be helpful. Some adults may be embarrassed or uncomfortable or may even find the process of obtaining the sputum to be nauseating. Provide reassurance and privacy to reduce their discomfort or embarrassment.

- Encourage the patient not to just spit into the cup. Explain that saliva and secretions from the nose are not the correct specimens.
- The best time of day to collect a sputum specimen is early morning before the patient brushes her teeth, uses mouthwash, or eats.

Objectives

Key Terms

Supplies/ Equipment

Pertinent Points

Age-Specific Considerations

Key Concepts

1. Wash hands.
2. Identify the correct patient.
3. Explain the procedure to the patient.
4. Assemble the equipment, and put on gloves.
5. Have the patient rinse out her mouth if she has eaten recently.
6. Ask the patient to take three or four deep breaths before coughing deeply from the lungs (Figure 4.3) and expectorating into the sputum cup.
7. Have the patient repeat step 6 until there is at least a table-spoon-size specimen. Provide the patient with tissues after she has produced the specimen.
8. Cover the specimen immediately, taking care not to touch the inside of the container.
9. Label the specimen immediately.
10. Document and report the results to the RN or preceptor.

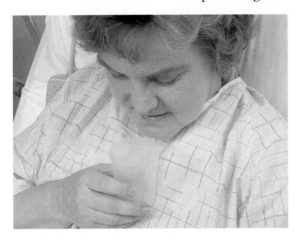

a

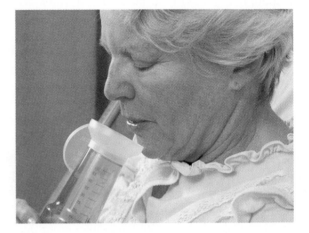

b

Figure 4.3 (a) Collecting a sterile sputum specimen, (b) an acid-fast bacilli sputum specimen for tuberculosis.

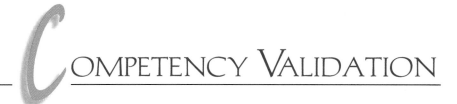

COMPETENCY VALIDATION

Skill: Obtaining a Sputum Specimen

Name _____

Preceptor _____

Date _____

Competency Statement   Obtains a sputum specimen while demonstrating correct sterile technique.

Not Competent: _____ 1. Is <u>unable to state reason</u> for task and <u>needs instructions</u> to perform task.

_____ 2. Understands reason for task but <u>needs instructions</u> to perform task.

Competent: _____ 3. Understands reason for task and is able to perform task but <u>needs to increase speed.</u>

_____ 4. Understands reason for task and is able to perform task <u>proficiently.</u>

Performance Criteria

The caregiver demonstrates the ability to do the following:

_____ 1. Wash hands.

_____ 2. Identify the correct patient.

_____ 3. Explain the procedure to the patient.

_____ 4. Assemble the equipment, and put on gloves.

_____ 5. Have the patient rinse out mouth if he or she has eaten recently.

_____ 6. Ask the patient to take three or four deep breaths before coughing deeply from the lungs before expectorating into the sputum cup.

_____ 7. Have the patient repeat step 6 until there is at least a tablespoon-size specimen. Provide the patient with tissues after he or she has produced the specimen.

_____ 8. Cover the specimen immediately, taking care not to touch the inside of the container.

_____ 9. Label the specimen immediately.

_____ 10. Document and report the results to the RN or preceptor.

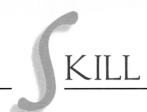

SKILL

Obtaining a Gastric Specimen

Purpose A patient may have a nasogastric tube inserted for a number of reasons: to empty the stomach (decompression), to feed the patient (gavage), to wash the lining of the stomach (lavage), or to obtain a specimen for gastric analysis. One type of gastric analysis is the method of measuring the pH of the secretions. If the secretions are acidic, it may indicate the overproduction of acid by the stomach. A high level of acid may lead to discomfort for the patient and potential irritation of the stomach. A physician will often order an antacid to be administered when pH levels fall too low (often for 4 and below).

Objectives

The caregiver demonstrates the ability to do the following:

1. Gather the correct supplies.

2. Communicate using a style that reduces the patient's anxiety.

3. Obtain a gastric specimen.

4. Apply the correct lab label.

5. Report the results of the procedure to the RN or preceptor.

Key Terms

Gastric Secretion The type of fluid found in the stomach.

Nasogastric Tube (NG Tube) A tube that is inserted into one of the nares of the nose and passed down the esophagus into the stomach.

pH A measure of how acidic or alkaline a fluid is. Water has a pH of 7. A pH of less than 7 is considered to be acidic, and a pH of more than 7 is considered to be alkaline.

Supplies/ Equipment

Gloves • 60-cc syringe • Nitrazine paper • Specimen cup

Pertinent Points

• Having a nasogastric tube in place is often uncomfortable for the patient.

• The patient may be alarmed at the thought of a caregiver doing something to the tube. Reassure the patient that the specimen collection process will not hurt.

• Explain all of your actions to the patient.

Age-Specific Considerations

Older adults or young children may require extra reassurance that the procedure will not cause them additional discomfort. When obtaining the specimen, avoid moving the nasogastric tube more than necessary. The skin of elderly individuals or anyone with skin sensitivity can be easily irritated by the tape and pressure of the tube on the nostrils.

Key Concept

*P*atients who have nasogastric tubes in place must remain with the head of the bed elevated at least 45 degrees. This prevents aspiration of gastric secretions into the lungs. Remember to maintain this positioning while obtaining the gastric specimen.

1. Wash hands.

2. Identify the correct patient.

3. Explain the procedure to the patient.

4. Assemble the equipment, and apply gloves.

5. Disconnect from suction source or unclamp the nasogastric tube.

6. Insert the syringe into the unclamped port of the nasogastric tube.

7. Withdraw approximately 10 cc of gastric secretions into the syringe (Figure 4.4).

8. Reclamp the nasogastric tube, or reconnect it to the wall suction, as ordered.

9. Empty the contents of the syringe into the specimen cup.

10. Dip the end of the Nitrazine paper into the gastric secretion. If Gastrocult or another commercial product is used, follow the directions provided.

11. Note the color that the Nitrazine paper changes to. Compare the paper's color to the colors on the Nitrazine container, and identify the closest color. This indicates the pH of the gastric secretions.

12. Document and report the level of the pH to the RN or preceptor, who will determine the need for any further action.

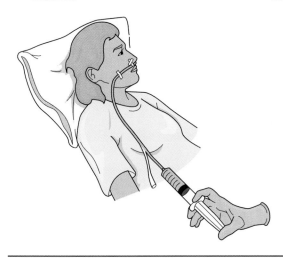

Figure 4.4 Collecting a gastric specimen from a nasogastric tube.

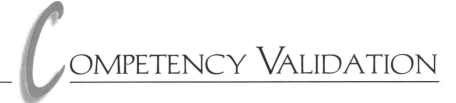

COMPETENCY VALIDATION

Skill: Obtaining a Gastric Specimen

Name _____

Preceptor _____

Date _____

Competency Statement   Demonstrates correct technique while obtaining a gastric specimen.

Not Competent: _____ 1. Is <u>unable to state reason</u> for task and <u>needs instructions</u> to perform task.

_____ 2. Understands reason for task but <u>needs instructions</u> to perform task.

Competent: _____ 3. Understands reason for task and is able to perform task but <u>needs to increase speed.</u>

_____ 4. Understands reason for task and is able to perform task <u>proficiently.</u>

Performance Criteria

The caregiver demonstrates the ability to do the following:

_____ 1. Wash hands.

_____ 2. Identify the correct patient.

_____ 3. Explain the procedure to the patient.

_____ 4. Assemble the equipment, and apply gloves.

_____ 5. Disconnect from suction source or unclamp the nasogastric tube.

_____ 6. Insert the syringe into the unclamped port of the nasogastric tube.

_____ 7. Withdraw approximately 10 cc of gastric secretions into the syringe.

_____ 8. Reclamp the nasogastric tube, or reconnect it to the wall suction, as ordered.

_____ 9. Empty the contents of the syringe into the specimen cup.

_____ 10. Dip the end of the Nitrazine paper into the gastric secretion.

_____ 11. Note the color that the Nitrazine paper changes to. Compare the paper's color to the colors on the Nitrazine container, and identify the closest color match. This indicates the pH of the gastric secretions.

_____ 12. Document and report the level of the pH to the RN or preceptor, who will determine the need for any further action.

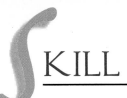

SKILL

Collecting Stool for Hemoccult Testing

Purpose Hemoccult testing allows for the quick detection of blood in stool. It is a noninvasive test for the patient. The presence of blood in stool may indicate many diseases and disorders. Hemoccult testing is often used to detect bleeding due to polyps or cancer of the intestinal tract.

The caregiver demonstrates the ability to do the following:

1. Gather the correct supplies.

2. Communicate using a style that reduces the patient's anxiety.

3. Obtain an adequate stool sample for Hemoccult testing.

4. Apply the correct lab label.

5. Perform Hemoccult test and read the result.

6. Report the results of the procedure to the RN or preceptor.

Objectives

Hemoccult Developer The solution that generates or triggers the chemical reaction to indicate the presence of blood.

Hemoccult Slide The paper slide used to test for the presence of blood in stool.

Gloves • Hemoccult slide • Applicator • Hemoccult developer • Lab label

- Correct identification of the patient and the specimen is crucial for the correct results and diagnosis.

- Explain the test to the patient.

- Assist the patient to have a bowel movement by helping him to a commode chair or onto a bedpan.

- Provide for privacy to help the patient relax.

Some teenagers or adults may be embarrassed to be asked to give a stool specimen. Provide privacy, and encourage them to try to have a bowel movement at their usual time.

Key Terms

Supplies/
Equipment

Pertinent
Points

Age-Specific
Considerations

Key Concepts

- The test results are most accurate when a clean bedpan is used to obtain the specimen.
- The patient should urinate before having a bowel movement to avoid mixing urine in the sample.
- Always wear vinyl or latex gloves when handling stool specimens.

1. Wash hands.
2. Identify the correct patient.
3. Explain the procedure to the patient.
4. Assemble the equipment, and put on gloves.
5. Label the Hemoccult slide with the patient's name, the date, and the address if applicable (Figure 4.5a).
6. Collect a small amount of stool on the applicator.
7. Apply the stool to the box marked "Box A" on the slide (Figure 4.5b).
8. From a different area of the stool, collect another small sample and apply it to the box marked "Box B" on the slide.
9. Close the cover of the slide, and secure.
10. Turn the slide over, and open the other cover.
11. Wait 3 to 5 minutes before applying two drops of developer over each stool smear (Figure 4.5c).
12. Apply one drop of developer to the "Performance Monitor" section.
13. Wait 60 seconds to read the result. If the stool sample turns a light blue color like the "(+)" section of the performance monitor, it is a positive result. If there is no change, it is a negative result.
14. Document and report the results to the RN or preceptor.

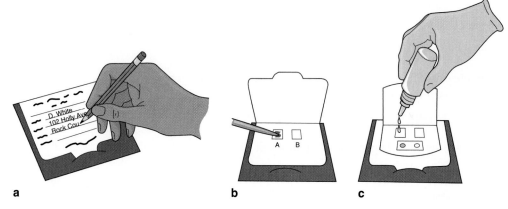

a   b   c

Figure 4.5 Testing stool specimen for occult blood.

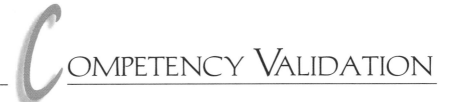

COMPETENCY VALIDATION

Skill: Collecting Stool for Hemoccult Testing

Name _____

Preceptor _____

Date _____

Competency Statement
Demonstrates correct technique to collect stool and perform Hemoccult testing.

Not Competent: _____ 1. Is <u>unable to state reason</u> for task and <u>needs instructions</u> to perform task.

_____ 2. Understands reason for task but <u>needs instructions</u> to perform task.

Competent: _____ 3. Understands reason for task and is able to perform task but <u>needs to increase speed.</u>

_____ 4. Understands reason for task and is able to perform task <u>proficiently.</u>

Performance Criteria

The caregiver demonstrates the ability to do the following:

_____ 1. Wash hands.

_____ 2. Identify the correct patient.

_____ 3. Explain the procedure to the patient.

_____ 4. Assemble the equipment, and apply gloves.

_____ 5. Label the Hemoccult slide with the patient's name, the date, and the address (if applicable).

_____ 6. Collect a small amount of stool on the applicator.

_____ 7. Apply the stool to the box marked "Box A" on the slide.

_____ 8. From a different area of the stool, collect another small sample and apply it to the box marked "Box B" on the slide.

_____ 9. Close the cover of the slide, and secure.

_____ 10. Turn the slide over, and open the other cover.

_____ 11. Wait 3 to 5 minutes before applying two drops of developer over each stool smear.

_____ 12. Apply one drop of developer to the "Performance Monitor" section.

_____ 13. Wait 60 seconds to read the result. If the stool sample turns a light blue color like the "(+)" section of the performance monitor, it is a positive result. If there is no change, it is a negative result.

_____ 14. Document and report the results to the RN or preceptor.

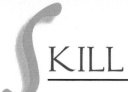

SKILL

Checking Blood Glucose

Purpose When a patient has diabetes or requires medications or treatments that may interfere with the body's ability to use insulin, it is important to monitor the level of the blood glucose. The most common method of testing blood glucose is with a blood glucose meter. Using a meter to determine when the blood glucose is high or low allows for early treatment with food or medication. There are many types of meters available. Learn about the type used by your institution or patient.

Objectives

The caregiver demonstrates the ability to do the following:

1. Gather the correct supplies.
2. Communicate using a style that reduces the patient's anxiety.
3. Prepare the blood glucose meter for a sample.
4. Obtain an adequate blood sample.
5. Record the results.
6. Report the results of the procedure to the RN or preceptor.

Key Terms

Diabetes Mellitus A disorder caused by the body's inability to convert sugar into energy due to inadequate insulin production or inadequate insulin usage.

Glucose Sugar.

Hyperglycemia Abnormally high blood glucose.

Hypoglycemia Abnormally low blood glucose.

Supplies/ Equipment

Gloves • Blood glucose meter • Test strips • Lancet • Disposable pipet • Small bandage

Pertinent Points

- Blood glucose monitoring allows for the early detection of hypoglycemia or hyperglycemia.
- The symptoms of hypoglycemia are excessive sweating, faintness, hunger, irritability, numbness of the tongue and lips, headache, trembling, and blurred vision.
- The symptoms of hyperglycemia are air hunger (heavy, labored breathing), loss of appetite, nausea, vomiting, weakness, abdominal pain, increased thirst, sweet fruity breath, increased urination, and dulled senses.
- If you note any of these symptoms or if the patient reports them to you, notify the nurse or preceptor immediately.

Age-Specific Considerations

Diabetes mellitus is a chronic disorder, and each patient will adjust to it in a unique way. Children may fear and dislike the intrusion of the needle pricks. Adolescents and adults may resent the intrusion as well as the lack of control that the disease creates. Adolescents may avoid following their treatment plans or diabetic diets because these things make them appear different from their friends. Adults and geriatric patients may fear potential complications or may be experiencing complications associated with diabetes.

*T*he primary use of blood glucose meters is to provide an accurate measure of the blood glucose, or blood sugar, level of diabetics. The goal is to keep the level as close to normal as possible. Medication and food requirements are influenced by the results of the test.

1. Wash hands.
2. Identify the correct patient and explain the procedure.
3. Assemble the equipment (Figure 4.6), and put on gloves.
4. Match the code on the test strips to the number on the meter. Check the expiration date on the test strips. Discard them if they have expired. The code number may have to be reset. Follow the meter's instructions.
5. Remove a test strip from the container, and then close it. Do not touch the white area on the strip.
6. Insert the lancet into the Penlet.
7. Place the end of the lancet firmly on the side of the patient's fingertip. Press the button on top of the Penlet.
8. Squeeze the finger gently to obtain a large drop of blood.
9. Slowly draw the blood up into the disposable pipet. Apply the blood

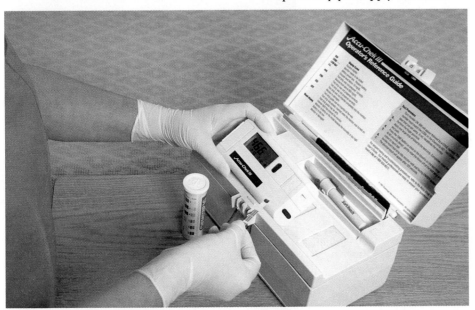

Figure 4.6 One of the many different devices available for monitoring blood glucose.

sample to the test strip. This prevents cross-contamination of body fluids between patients. An alternative is to drop the blood directly onto the test strip if the machine is used for only one patient (Figures 4.7 and 4.8).

10. Wait the indicated amount of time for the results to appear on the meter (Figure 4.9).

11. Apply a bandage to the patient's finger.

12. Clean and dispose of the equipment as necessary.

13. Document and report the results to the RN or preceptor.

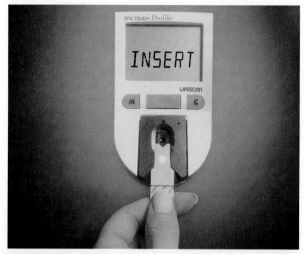

Figure 4.7 Inserting a test strip into the machine. (Photo courtesy of Johnson & Johnson.)

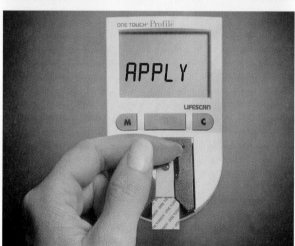

Figure 4.8 Applying a drop of blood directly onto the test strip. (Photo courtesy of Johnson & Johnson.)

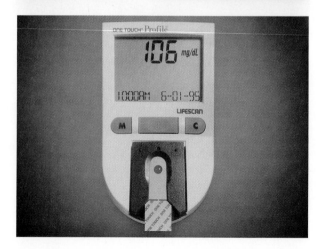

Figure 4.9 Reading the result. (Photo courtesy of Johnson & Johnson.)

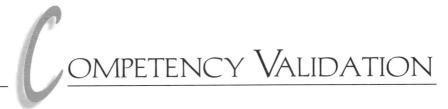

COMPETENCY VALIDATION

Name _____

Preceptor _____

Date _____

Competency Statement   Demonstrate correct sterile technique while checking blood glucose.

Not Competent: _____ 1. Is <u>unable to state reason</u> for task and <u>needs instructions</u> to perform task.

_____ 2. Understands reason for task but <u>needs instructions</u> to perform task.

Competent: _____ 3. Understands reason for task and is able to perform task but <u>needs to increase speed.</u>

_____ 4. Understands reason for task and is able to perform task <u>proficiently.</u>

Performance Criteria

The caregiver demonstrates the ability to do the following:

_____ 1. Wash hands.

_____ 2. Identify the correct patient and explain the procedure.

_____ 3. Assemble the equipment, and apply gloves.

_____ 4. Match the code on the test strips to the number on the meter. Check the expiration date on the test strips. Discard them if they have expired. The code number may have to be reset. Follow the meter's instructions.

_____ 5. Remove a test strip from the container, and then close it. Do not touch the white area on the strip.

_____ 6. Insert the lancet into the Penlet.

_____ 7. Place the end of the lancet firmly on the side of the patient's fingertip. Press button on the top of the Penlet.

_____ 8. Squeeze the finger gently to obtain a large drop of blood.

_____ 9. Slowly draw the blood up into the disposable pipet. Apply the blood sample to the test strip. This prevents cross-contamination of body fluids between patients. An alternative is to drop the blood directly onto the test strip if the machine is used for only one patient.

_____ 10. Wait the indicated amount of time for the results to appear on the meter.

_____ 11. Apply a bandage to the patient's finger.

_____ 12. Clean and dispose of the equipment as necessary.

_____ 13. Document and report the results to the RN or preceptor.

CHAPTER 5
PHLEBOTOMY AND IV THERAPY

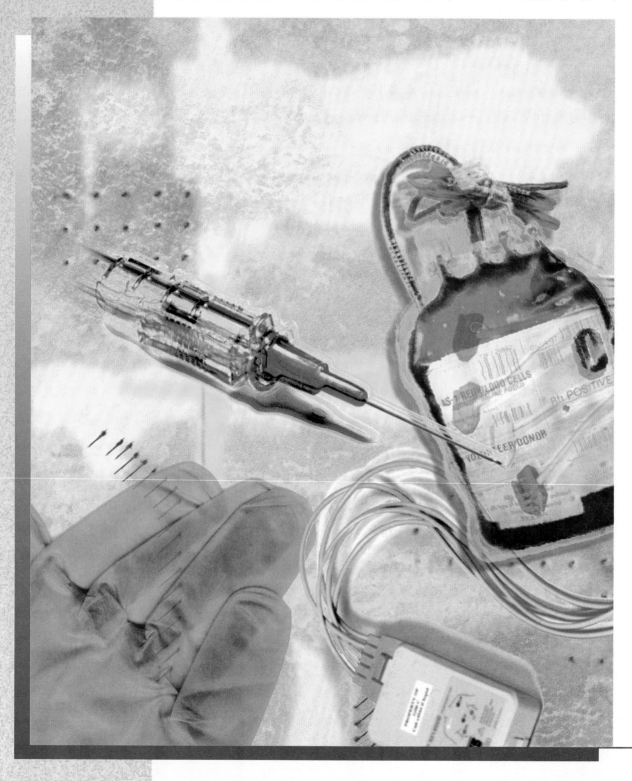

*C*aregivers often encounter patients who must have their blood drawn for various tests. Collecting blood specimens for laboratory testing allows physicians and caregivers to identify the patient's status, confirm a diagnosis, or assess the extent of the patient's disease. Physicians will determine treatment plans or order medications based on the test results. IV lines have become so commonplace that most hospitalized patients have one in place. Health care has evolved to the point that some patients are discharged with an IV in place so they can continue to receive IV antibiotics, chemotherapy, or pain medications in their home. Caregivers need to frequently assess the IV site as complications may occur that require interventions.

This chapter includes information on selecting veins and recognizing problems in IV therapy. In addition, it prepares caregivers to perform the following skills, which are listed under the relevant section titles:

Phlebotomy

Blood Specimen Collection

Obtaining Blood Cultures

Using a Lancet or a Microlance for a Microdraw or an Infant Heel Stick

Measuring Bleeding Time

IV Therapy

Inserting a Heplock

Inserting a Butterfly (Winged Infusion Device)

Inserting a Peripheral IV in an Adult

Inserting a Peripheral IV in a Child

Recognizing Problems in IV Therapy

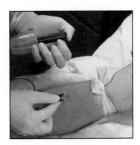
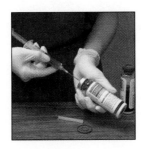
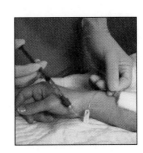

Phlebotomy

Selecting a Vein

Determining which vein to use is one of the primary considerations to be taken into account before starting an IV. In a young, healthy adult, there is often an abundance of peripheral hand and arm veins to choose from. Unfortunately, this is not usually the case. Age, illness, previous therapies, and other factors frequently limit the number of veins from which a caregiver will have to choose.

Adult

In reviewing the hand and arm veins from distal to proximal (from the fingers toward the shoulder), first the veins of the fingers, or the *digital* veins, are found (Figure 5.1). These veins are located along the lateral (side) and dorsal (top) portions of the fingers. The catheter of choice for use in these veins is a small-gauge (22-gauge) catheter that can be anchored securely in this area. A padded tongue blade can be used to splint the finger and prevent dislodging. The veins of the fingers are usually not the best choice when starting an IV. They are generally smaller than the veins of the forearm and therefore provide less hemodilution and a greater likelihood that phlebitis will occur.

Next are the three *metacarpal* veins, which are located on the back of each hand and begin at the junction of the digital veins (Figure 5.1). The catheter of choice for these veins is usually a 22- or 20-gauge catheter. Use a short catheter, ¾ or 1 inch in length, to prevent catheter flexion as the joints of the hand and wrist are moved. A flexible catheter should be used instead of a metal needle, if possible, when using the finger or hand veins for IV therapy. This area has many joints, and a metal needle could easily become dislodged from the vein if not immobi-

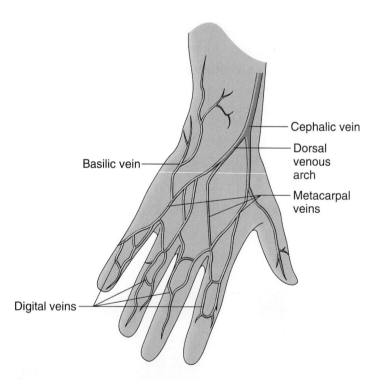

Figure 5.1 Superficial veins of the fingers and hand.

lized by an arm board. Because of restriction of movement and limited size, the veins of the fingers and hand are not normally the first choice for long-term or irritating therapies.

The veins of the forearm are usually the veins of choice in selecting a site for IV placement in an adult. These veins are usually larger, straighter, and more easily secured than the veins of the fingers and hands. The long bones of the arm serve as natural arm boards, and the flat surfaces of the forearm allow the IV to be more easily secured with less loss of mobility for the patient (Figure 5.2).

The *cephalic* vein originates from the metacarpal veins near the base of the thumb and travels along the radial bone of the forearm. This vein is often referred to as the intern's friend because of its prominence and relative ease of accessibility. The *basilic* vein originates from the metacarpal veins on the opposite side of the hand. It follows the course of the ulnar bone up to the elbow and then travels along the inner aspect of the upper arm, where it joins the cephalic vein at the axillary vein near the shoulder.

Both the cephalic and basilic veins of the forearm, along with the median basilic and accessory cephalic veins, are good choices for IV therapy. Catheters or needles from 22 to 18 gauge are normally used. Because these veins have a tendency to roll, secure traction is required to increase the success of the IV start.

Begin IV therapy at the most distal vein that can be palpated. Subsequent venipunctures should be proximal to the last venipuncture site. Remember, if a vein has chemical phlebitis (an irritation from medications infused) and you start an IV distal to that site, the irritating substance may continue to flow through that vein toward the heart, thereby worsening the phlebitis.

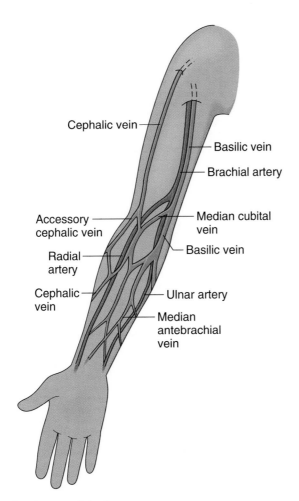

Figure 5.2 Superficial veins of the forearm.

The *antecubital* veins, located at the inner aspect of the elbow, are a good choice in emergency situations and are the veins of choice for blood drawing. All sizes of catheter are acceptable, especially large 18- or 16-gauge catheters for rapid infusion of fluids or blood products. This site is usually uncomfortable for the patient because flexion of the elbow must be prevented in order for the IV to flow properly. If this site is used in an emergency, it is preferable to change the site within 24 hours if possible.

Infant and Child

Depending on the child's age, it is usually more difficult to find an appropriate site for IV therapy in a pediatric patient than in an adult. IVs are frequently started in the hand, forearm, antecubital fossa, and upper arm. As these are considered to be the preferred sites, they should be used or evaluated first. The foot and lower leg are normally reserved for children below walking age.

The veins of the hand include the digital and metacarpal veins. The forearm veins commonly used are the supplementary cephalic, the basilic, and the median antecubital. The upper arm contains the basilic and the cephalic veins. The main veins of the foot and leg are the greater and lesser *saphenous* veins.

Less optimal sites for IVs in children include the wrist, abdomen, axilla, and knee. These are usually only considered in infants or very small children. These sites should be considered only when the above sites are not available. Infiltration in any of these sites may cause nerve or tissue damage.

The scalp is another site that is often used in infants up to 12 to 18 months of age. The scalp has many superficial veins, including the *frontal* or *metopic,* the *superior temporal,* the *occipital,* and the *posterior auricular* veins. Care must be taken to distinguish these veins from arteries in the scalp (Figure 5.3).

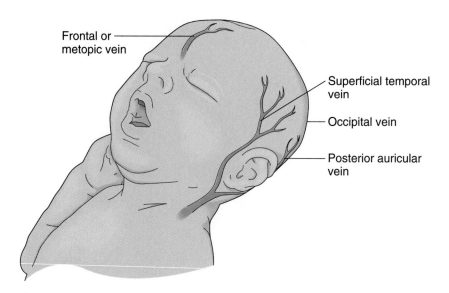

Figure 5.3 Sites for infant scalp vein infusions.

Key Information

If an artery is accidentally used—as indicated by bright red, pulsating blood return—the IV should be removed immediately and pressure held on the site until the bleeding stops. A pressure bandage should be applied and kept in place for 30 minutes. When an artery is accidentally punctured, many facilities require that an incident report be completed and a supervisor, physician, or pathologist notified.

Care must be taken to prepare the infant's parents before they see the child; the sight of an IV placed in an infant's head can be distressing. The child's hair might need to be shaved or clipped. Remove the smallest amount of hair necessary to achieve a clear site and to affix the IV securely. Figure 5.4 shows how a rubber band may be used as a tourniquet on the baby's scalp.

Small-gauge, thin-walled over-the-needle catheters are usually preferred to winged, metal needles in children and infants. Usually, 24- to 22-gauge catheters are used in infants and children. Catheters as small as 26 gauge may be used for therapy in neonates.

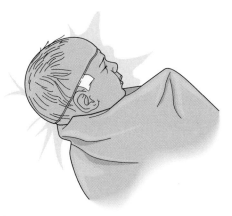

Figure 5.4 Applying a tourniquet on an infant head.

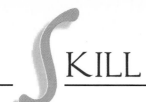 SKILL

Blood Specimen Collection

Purpose Blood, which flows through both the patient's arteries and veins, is usually drawn from peripheral veins in the patient's arms or hands to be tested for many things. Physicians order blood tests to measure electrolyte balance, abnormal functioning of body organs, blood counts, bacterial invasion, and other things that assist them in diagnosing and treating illness.

Objectives

The caregiver demonstrates the ability to do the following:

1. Gather the correct supplies.

2. Communicate using a style that reduces the patient's anxiety.

3. Maintain sterile technique and use standard precautions.

4. Identify the correct colored tubes to be used for each test that the doctor has ordered.

5. Correctly perform the venipuncture.

6. Draw blood in the appropriate order related to the color of the blood tube.

7. Apply pressure and place a sterile bandage over the venipuncture site.

8. Dispose of the needle in a sharps container.

9. Correctly label the blood tubes.

10. Arrange for the blood to be taken to the laboratory.

11. Report the results of the procedure to the RN or preceptor.

Key Terms

Uncoagulated Blood Blood that is collected in a tube and mixed with an anticoagulant so it does not clot. This allows the blood specimen to be tested in a liquid form with the cells in suspension.

Coagulated Blood Blood that is collected in a tube and allowed to clot. As the blood stands, a clear liquid, called serum, separates from the clotted blood cells.

Hematoma An accumulation of blood beneath the skin that results in a discoloration of the skin. Also called a bruise.

Peripheral Vein Surface vein that can be used as a site for venipuncture.

Supplies/ Equipment

Vacutainer system with appropriate tubes, needle, and holder • Tourniquet • Clean disposable gloves • Alcohol swabs • Sterile gauze • Sterile adhesive bandage

Pertinent Points

- A physician's order is required for obtaining a blood specimen.

- Patients are often anxious about being stuck by a needle and about the amount of blood to be taken.

- A confident attitude and a reassuring manner will serve to calm patients and gain their cooperation. If the patient expresses concern, explain that relatively little blood will be taken. Explain also that there will be some discomfort during the procedure but that if the patient holds very still, the discomfort will be minimized.

- Observe the puncture site for swelling or hematoma during and after the venipuncture. Discontinue venipuncture if a hematoma forms. Apply gentle pressure over the venipuncture site for 2 to 3 minutes. If the patient is on anticoagulant therapy, apply gentle pressure for up to 5 minutes to prevent bleeding.
- If you cannot obtain the sample within two venipunctures or if you cannot find an appropriate vein to stick, notify the RN immediately. Do not stick a patient more than twice.
- Unacceptable sites for blood collection include arteries, heparin locks, fistulas, shunts, bovine or Gortex grafts, foot and leg veins, hematomas, mastectomy sites, above an IV site, scarred or burned areas, and edematous areas.

Age-Specific Considerations

Patients of any age might have a fear of needles. Explain what you are going to do before beginning the procedure. Assess the patient's ability to immobilize the limb that you are sticking. Children and confused individuals of any age might need to be physically restrained to prevent movement when the needle is in the skin.

One of the most important things for improving success in venipuncture in children is to prevent movement of the selected site. Always try to have another caregiver assist with immobilization. Parents are usually not ideal for this purpose because they are not always able to continue to hold their children as they become upset or cry in pain.

Key Concepts

- Check the patient's name or armband for positive identification.
- Do not attempt to stick a patient more than twice. Have another caregiver attempt the draw.
- Never attempt a venipuncture without feeling or seeing a vein.
- Do not keep the tourniquet on the patient's arm for more than 2 minutes.
- Do not prelabel tubes. Initial requisition slips only after the specimen has been collected.
- Use standard precautions, and follow all agency policies and procedures.
- Discard needles only in the appropriate boxes or containers.
- Never draw a blood speciman above an IV site.

Steps

1. Wash hands.
2. Assemble the equipment (Figure 5.5a).
3. Identify the correct patient.
4. Explain the procedure to the patient, emphasizing the need to hold the selected arm as still as possible.
5. Put on gloves.
6. Attach the needle to the Vacutainer holder (Figure 5.5b).
7. Select the correct tubes for the blood samples you are going to draw.
8. Insert one tube into the holder, and push the tube stopper partway into the needle. (Tubes without anticoagulants are always filled before those with anticoagulants.)
9. Apply the tourniquet 3 to 4 inches above the elbow.
10. Select a site for venipuncture. Assess the antecubital space of both arms to locate the best site (Figures 5.5c and d).
11. Clean the venipuncture site with an alcohol swab (Figure 5.5e). Allow to dry for several seconds. Do not touch the site after cleaning.
12. Remove the needle cover.
13. Use nondominant hand to secure and stretch the skin below the site. This stabilizes the vein and prevents it from rolling.
14. Carefully insert the needle through the skin, bevel up, in one fluid motion (Figure 5.5f).

15. Secure the Vacutainer holder with one hand while firmly pushing the tube into the holder with the thumb of the other hand (Figure 5.5g). When the tube is full, withdraw it (Figure 5.5h). If the blood specimen tube has additives, gently invert it eight to ten times to mix the additive with the blood. Insert the next tube into the holder, and repeat the process until all of the required samples have been drawn.

16. Release the tourniquet.

17. Place sterile gauze over the venipuncture site, and withdraw the needle from the skin (Figure 5.5i).

18. Apply pressure to the site for 2 to 3 minutes. (More time might be needed for patients who are on anticoagulant therapy.)

19. Discard the needle in a sharps container (Figure 5.5j).

20. Apply a sterile adhesive bandage to the site (Figure 5.5k).

21. Clean the area, and dispose of the waste in accordance with the facility's policy.

22. Label the tubes with the patient's name, the date and time, and your initials.

23. Finish filling out the requisitions (Figure 5.5l).

24. Remove and discard gloves; wash hands.

25. Ensure that the blood samples and requisitions are delivered to the proper laboratory for testing.

26. Document and report the results to the RN or preceptor.

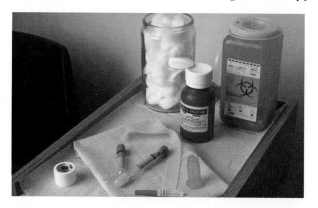

a

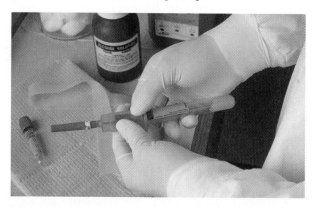

b

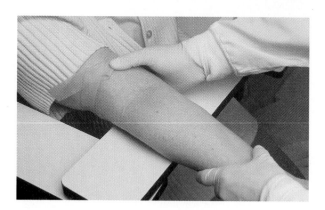

c

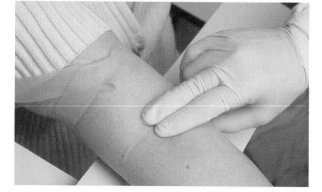

d

Figure 5.5 Using a Vacutainer to draw blood.

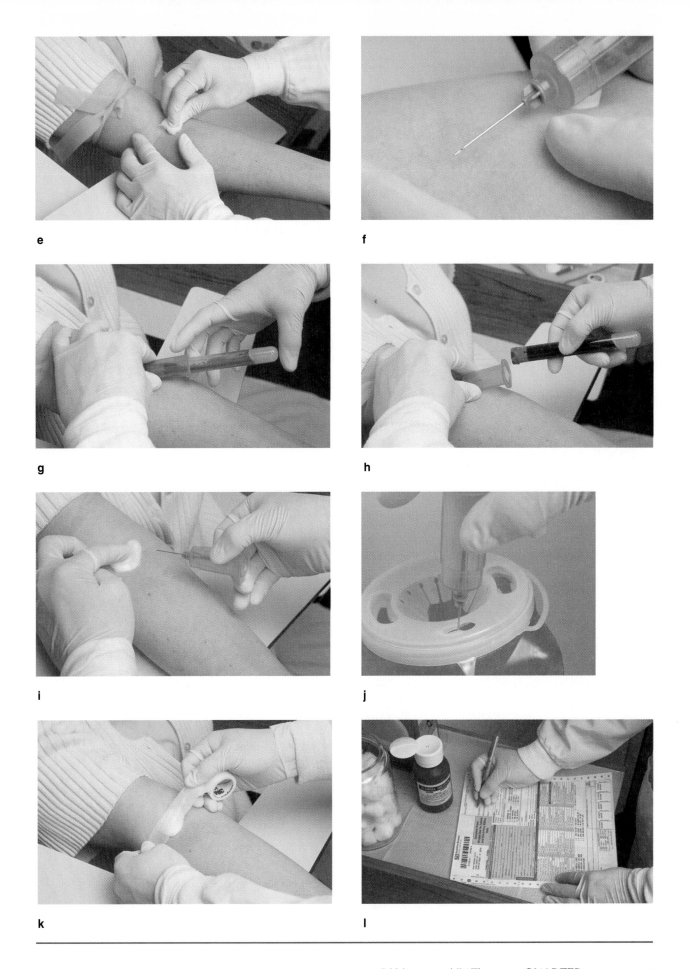

e

f

g

h

i

j

k

l

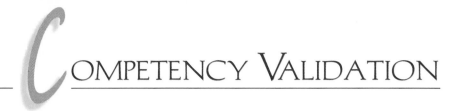

COMPETENCY VALIDATION

Name _____

Preceptor _____

Date _____

Competency Statement Draws blood while demonstrating correct sterile technique.

Not Competent: _____ 1. Is <u>unable to state reason</u> for task and <u>needs instructions</u> to perform task.

_____ 2. Understands reason for task but <u>needs instructions</u> to perform task.

Competent: _____ 3. Understands reason for task and is able to perform task but <u>needs to increase speed.</u>

_____ 4. Understands reason for task and is able to perform task <u>proficiently.</u>

Performance Criteria

The caregiver demonstrates the ability to do the following:

_____ 1. Wash hands.

_____ 2. Assemble the equipment.

_____ 3. Identify the correct patient.

_____ 4. Explain the procedure to the patient, emphasizing the need to hold the selected arm as still as possible.

_____ 5. Put on gloves.

_____ 6. Attach the needle to the Vacutainer holder.

_____ 7. Select the correct tubes for the blood samples you are going to draw.

_____ 8. Insert one tube into the holder, and push the tube stopper partway into the needle. (Tubes without antico-agulants are always filled before those with anticoagulants.)

_____ 9. Apply the tourniquet 3 to 4 inches above the elbow.

_____ 10. Select a site for venipuncture. Assess the antecubital space of both arms to locate the best site.

_____ 11. Clean the venipuncture site with an alcohol swab. Allow to dry for several seconds. Do not touch the site after cleaning.

_____ 12. Remove the needle cover.

_____ 13. Use nondominant hand to secure and stretch the skin below the site. This stabilizes the vein and prevents it from rolling.

_____ 14. Carefully insert the needle through the skin, bevel up, in one fluid motion.

_____ 15. Secure the vacutainer holder with one hand while firmly pushing the tube into the holder with the thumb of the other hand. When the tube is full, withdraw it. If the blood specimen tube has additives, gently invert it eight to ten times to mix the additive with the blood. Insert the next tube into the holder, and repeat the process until all of the required samples have been drawn.

_____ 16. Release the tourniquet.

_____ 17. Place sterile gauze over the venipuncture site, and withdraw the needle from the skin.

_____ 18. Apply pressure to the site for 2 to 3 minutes. (More time might be needed for patients who are on anticoagulant therapy.)

_____ 19. Discard the needle in a sharps container.

_____ 20. Apply a sterile adhesive bandage to the site.

_____ 21. Clean the area, and dispose of the waste in accordance with the facility's policy.

_____ 22. Label the tubes with the patient's name, the date and time, and your initials.

_____ 23. Finish filling out the requisitions.

_____ 24. Remove and discard gloves; wash hands.

_____ 25. Ensure that the blood samples and requisitions are delivered to the proper laboratory for testing.

_____ 26. Document and report the results to the RN or preceptor.

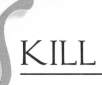KILL

Obtaining Blood Cultures

Purpose   When a patient is suspected to have a septicemia, blood cultures are obtained to identify the causative microorganisms. Blood cultures are drawn when a patient is feverish or having chills with a spiking fever. Blood cultures are usually ordered in sets (one aerobic and one anaerobic), which are usually drawn from more than one venipuncture site, often spaced over a period of time.

Objectives

The caregiver demonstrates the ability to do the following:

1. Gather the correct supplies.

2. Communicate using a style that reduces the patient's anxiety.

3. Maintain sterile technique and use standard precautions.

4. Correctly identify aerobic and anaerobic blood culture bottles.

5. Correctly prep the venipuncture site and the blood culture bottle tops.

6. Correctly perform the venipuncture.

7. Inject the blood into the blood culture bottles using sterile technique.

8. Apply pressure and place a sterile bandage over the venipuncture site.

9. Dispose of the needle in a sharps container.

10. Correctly label the blood culture bottles.

11. Arrange for the blood to be taken to the laboratory.

12. Report the results of the procedure to the RN or preceptor.

Key Terms

Aerobic Able to live only in the presence of free oxygen.

Anaerobic Able to live without air, like some microbes.

Septicemia An infection in the blood; the absorption of pathologic organisms into the blood, where they multiply rapidly.

Supplies/ Equipment

2 needles • 20-cc syringe • Blood culture bottles • Povidone-iodine swabs • Sterile gauze • Tourniquet • Sterile disposable gloves • Sterile adhesive bandage • Alcohol pad or wipe

Pertinent Points

- A physician's order is required for obtaining a blood culture.

- Patients are often anxious about being stuck by a needle. A confident attitude and a reassuring manner will serve to calm patients and gain their cooperation. Explain that there will be some discomfort during the procedure but that if the patient holds very still, the discomfort will be minimized.

- Observe the puncture site for swelling or hematoma during and after the venipuncture. Apply gentle pressure over the venipuncture site for 2 to 3 minutes.

Age-Specific Considerations

Patients of any age might have a fear of needles. Explain what you are going to do before beginning the procedure. Assess the patient's ability to immobilize the limb that you are sticking. Children and confused individuals of any age might need to be physically restrained to prevent movement when the needle is in the skin. This is especially important in drawing blood cultures because of the necessity for strict asepsis in getting the blood into the culture bottle.

- Extreme care must be taken in preparing the skin and in preventing contamination during the procedure. Contamination of the blood culture by bacteria on the skin can cause an incorrect diagnosis of infection or a delay in treatment while the blood culture is repeated to verify the results.
- If you cannot obtain the sample within two venipunctures or if you cannot find an appropriate vein to stick, notify the RN immediately. Do not stick a patient more than twice.
- Never draw blood cultures above on IV site.

Steps

1. Wash hands.
2. Assemble the equipment.
3. Identify the correct patient.
4. Explain the procedure to the patient, emphasizing the need to hold the selected arm as still as possible to prevent failed venipuncture or contamination.
5. Attach a needle to the 20-cc syringe.
6. Prepare the blood culture bottles by removing the cap from the rubber diaphragm and cleaning the diaphragm thoroughly with an alcohol pad. Allow to dry.
7. Apply the tourniquet 3 to 4 inches above the elbow.
8. Select a site for venipuncture. Assess the antecubital space of both arms to locate the best site.
9. Put on gloves.
10. Clean the venipuncture site with an alcohol pad or povidone-iodine swab. Using a circular motion, start from the venipuncture site and continue outward approximately 3 inches. Repeat twice. Allow to dry. Do not touch the site after cleaning.

11. Remove the needle cover.
12. Use nondominant hand to secure and stretch the skin below the site. This stabilizes the vein and prevents it from rolling.
13. Carefully insert the needle through the skin, bevel up, in one fluid motion.
14. When the vein has been entered and blood return is obtained, slowly pull back the plunger and withdraw 20-cc of blood or use a blood culture adaptor (Figure 5.6a).
15. Release the tourniquet.
16. Place sterile gauze over the venipuncture site, and withdraw the needle from the skin.
17. Apply pressure to the site for 2 to 3 minutes. (More time might be needed for patients who are on anticoagulant therapy.)
18. Change the needle, and inject 10 cc of blood through the diaphragm of the anaerobic bottle. Next place 10 cc of blood in the aerobic bottle. Try not to inject air into either bottle; this is especially important in the anaerobic bottle (Figure 5.6b).

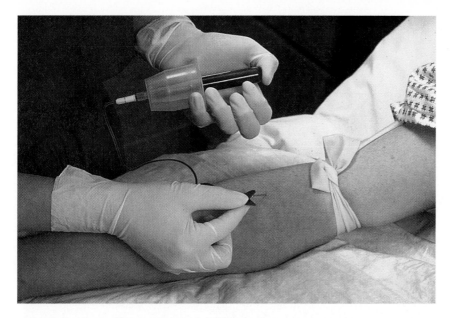

a

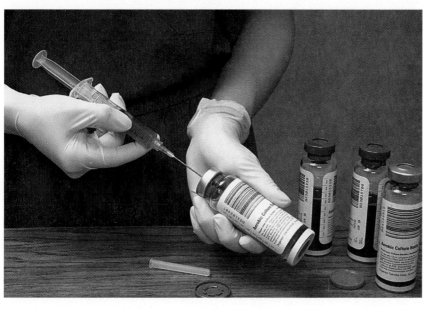

b

Figure 5.6 a. caregiver withdraws the patient's blood for blood cultures using a blood culture adaptor or syringe. **b.** Injecting 10 cc of blood in the aerobic bottle.

19. Discard the needles in a sharps container.

20. Apply a sterile adhesive bandage to the site.

21. Clean the area, and dispose of the waste in accordance with the facility's policy.

22. Label the bottles with the patient's name, the date and time, and your initials.

23. Remove and discard gloves; wash hands.

24. Finish filling out the requisitions.

25. Ensure that the blood cultures and the requisitions are delivered to the proper laboratory for testing.

26. Document and report the results to the RN or preceptor.

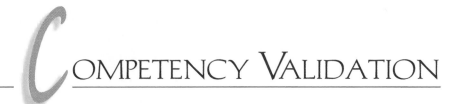

COMPETENCY VALIDATION

Skill: Obtaining Blood Cultures

Name _____

Preceptor _____

Date _____

Competency Statement Obtains blood cultures while demonstrating correct sterile technique.

Not Competent: _____ 1. Is <u>unable to state reason</u> for task and <u>needs instructions</u> to perform task.

_____ 2. Understands reason for task but <u>needs instructions</u> to perform task.

Competent: _____ 3. Understands reason for task and is able to perform task but <u>needs to increase speed.</u>

_____ 4. Understands reason for task and is able to perform task <u>proficiently.</u>

Performance Criteria

The caregiver demonstrates the ability to do the following:

_____ 1. Wash hands.

_____ 2. Assemble the equipment.

_____ 3. Identify the correct patient.

_____ 4. Explain the procedure to the patient, emphasizing the need to hold the selected arm as still as possible to prevent failed venipuncture or contamination.

_____ 5. Attach a needle to the 20-cc syringe or blood culture adaptor.

_____ 6. Prepare the blood culture bottles by removing the cap from the rubber diaphragm and cleaning the diaphragm thoroughly with povidone-iodine. Allow to dry.

_____ 7. Apply the tourniquet 3 to 4 inches above the elbow.

_____ 8. Select a site for venipuncture. Assess the antecubital space of both arms to locate the best site.

_____ 9. Put on gloves.

_____ 10. Clean the venipuncture site with a povidone-iodine swab. Using a circular motion, start from the venipuncture site and continue outward approximately 3 inches. Repeat twice. Allow to dry. Do not touch the site after cleaning.

_____ 11. Remove the needle cover.

_____ 12. Use nondominant hand to secure and stretch the skin below the site. This stabilizes the vein and prevents it from rolling.

_____ 13. Carefully insert the needle through the skin, bevel up, in one fluid motion.

_____ 14. When the vein has been entered and blood return is obtained, slowly pull back the plunger and withdraw 20 cc of blood. An alternative method is to attach the adaptor to the blood culture bottle.

_____ 15. Release the tourniquet.

_____ 16. Place sterile gauze over the venipuncture site, and withdraw the needle from the skin.

_____ 17. Apply pressure to the site for 2 to 3 minutes. (More time might be needed for patients who are on anticoagulant therapy.)

_____ 18. Change the needle, and inject 10 cc of blood through the diaphragm of the anaerobic bottle. Next place 10 cc of blood in the aerobic bottle. Try not to inject air into either bottle; this is especially important in the anaerobic bottle.

_____ 19. Discard the needles in a sharps container.

_____ 20. Apply a sterile adhesive bandage to the site.

_____ 21. Clean the area, and dispose of the waste in accordance with the facility's policy.

_____ 22. Label the bottles with the patient's name, the date and time, and your initials.

_____ 23. Remove and discard gloves; wash hands.

_____ 24. Finish filling out the requisitions.

_____ 25. Ensure that the blood cultures and the requisitions are delivered to the proper laboratory for testing.

_____ 26. Document and report the results to the RN or preceptor.

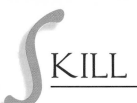

SKILL

Using a Lancet or a Microlance for a Microdraw or an Infant Heel Stick

Purpose Microdraw, or skin puncture, is used to collect blood specimens from patients of all ages. Although small in size, these specimens are adequate for many laboratory tests. Blood collected from a skin puncture is a mixture of arterial, venous, and capillary blood. Lancets are used to collect blood from toddlers through adults. Microlances or safety flow lancets are used when performing an infant heel stick.

The caregiver demonstrates the ability to do the following:

1. Gather the correct supplies.

2. Communicate using a style that reduces the patient's anxiety. Or explain procedure to the parent or guardian.

3. Maintain sterile technique.

4. Follow standard precautions.

5. Correctly prep the site.

6. Identify acceptable sites for skin puncture.

7. Collect the blood sample using the microdraw technique.

8. Apply pressure and place a sterile bandage over the site.

9. Dispose of the lancet in the sharps container.

10. Correctly label the blood sample.

11. Arrange for the blood to be taken to the laboratory.

12. Report the results of the procedure to the RN or preceptor.

Objectives

Lancet A small, extremely sharp, individually wrapped, single-use sterile, metal, or plastic object used to puncture the skin, cut the capillaries, and cause bleeding at the puncture site. Lancets come in two sizes: 2.4 mm (short-point or microlance) for use with infants or small children and 5.0 mm (long point) for adult use.

Microvette Collector A preassembled system containing a capillary unit and a graduated collection tube with an attached stopper. Microvette collectors are available with or without anticoagulants and with a serum separator gel.

Key Terms

Alcohol swab • Blood-collecting equipment • Clean gloves • Dry gauze pads • Spot adhesive bandage • Sterile disposable lancets

Supplies/ Equipment

• Unless there is a specific physician's order, the caregiver chooses the site for the collection of skin puncture specimens. These specimens may be obtained from the most medial or lateral portions of the plantar heel surface or the big toe in an infant or child under age 1 (Figure 5.7a).

• The sides of the middle and fourth fingers are the common sites for older children and adults (Figure 5.7b).

• A warm cloth can be applied to the selected site for a few minutes before sticking the site. This helps promote blood flow to the site.

Pertinent Points

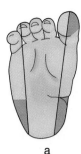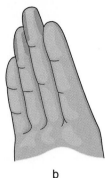

Figure 5.7 Acceptable sites for skin puncture (shaded areas).

a   b

- There are two types of microvette collectors. Microvettes with a purple cap contain powdered EDTA, are used for CBCs, and will collect up to 1 milliliter of blood. To ensure proper mixing, microvettes with anticoagulants should not be filled beyond 500 ul. Blood platelets have a tendency to clump; therefore hematology specimens should be collected first. Microvettes with a red cap are available in two types, either a plain interior or with a serum separator with gel.

Age-Specific Considerations

Patients of all ages might benefit from microdraw, or skin puncture, as only a very small amount of blood is needed. In ambulatory or outpatient settings, it can be helpful to have a parent in the room during the procedure to comfort the infant. If the parent is upset about the procedure or is uncomfortable with the sight of blood, another caregiver should hold the child. Explain the procedure to the infant's parents before beginning the procedure to alleviate some of their concerns.

Key Concept

*A*void using sites that are swollen or edematous or have previously been used.

Steps

1. Wash hands.
2. Assemble the equipment.
   a. Clean gloves
   b. Alcohol swab
   c. Safety flow lancet
   d. Capillary tubes
   e. Blood label
   f. Adhesive bandage
3. Identify the correct patient.
4. Explain the procedure to the patient, parent, or guardian, emphasizing the need to hold the selected finger (adult) or foot (infant) as still as possible.
5. Put on gloves.
6. Identify acceptable sites for skin puncture. Avoid sites that are swollen or edematous or have previously been used. Clean the selected site with an alcohol swab.
7. Hold the lancet at a 45-degree angle to the surface to be punctured. Do not direct the lancet toward a bone (Figure 5.8).
8. Wipe away the first drops of blood. Collect the blood sample by gently squeezing the heel and allowing the blood to flow into the tube.

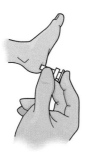
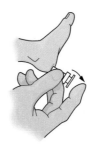
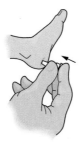
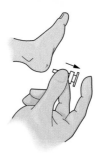

Hold lancet on site with moderate pressure.

Depress plunger with index finger to make puncture.

Immediately release plunger while holding lancet on site.

Remove lancet.

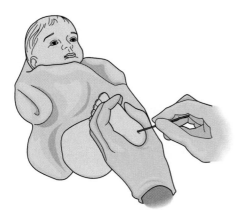
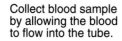

Collect blood sample by allowing the blood to flow into the tube.

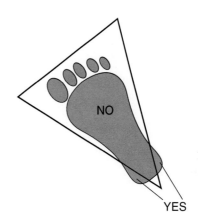

Figure 5.8 Using a safety flow lancet for an infant microdraw.

9. Apply adhesive bandage to puncture site.

10. Discard the lancet in a sharps container.

11. Correctly label the blood sample with patient name, date, and your initials.

12. Remove and discard gloves; wash hands.

13. Ensure that the blood sample is delivered to the proper laboratory for testing.

14. Document or notify the RN/preceptor that the blood sample has been obtained.

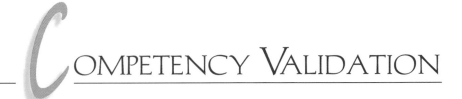

COMPETENCY VALIDATION

Skill: Performing a Microdraw Using a Microlance-Infant Heel Stick

Name _____

Preceptor _____

Date _____

Competency Statement

Performs an infant heel stick (microdraw) while demonstrating correct sterile technique.

Not Competent: _____ 1. Is <u>unable to state reason</u> for task and <u>needs instructions</u> to perform task.

_____ 2. Understands reason for task but <u>needs instructions</u> to perform task.

Competent: _____ 3. Understands reason for task and is able to perform task but <u>needs to increase speed.</u>

_____ 4. Understands reason for task and is able to perform task <u>proficiently.</u>

Performance Criteria

The caregiver demonstrates the ability to do the following:

_____ 1. Wash hands.

_____ 2. Assemble the equipment.
   a. clean gloves
   b. alcohol swab
   c. safety flow lancet
   d. capillary tube
   e. adhesive bandage
   f. blood label

_____ 3. Identify the correct patient.

_____ 4. Explain the procedure to the parent or guardian, emphasizing the need to hold the selected foot as still as possible.

_____ 5. Put on gloves.

_____ 6. Identify acceptable sites for skin puncture. Avoid sites that are swollen or edematous or have previously been used. Clean the selected site with an alcohol swab.

_____ 7. Hold the safety flow lancet at a 45-degree angle to the surface to be punctured. Do not direct the microlance toward a bone.

_____ 8. Wipe away the first drops of blood. Collect the blood sample using the microdraw technique.

_____ 9. Apply adhesive bandage to puncture site.

_____ 10. Discard the lancet in a sharps container.

_____ 11. Correctly label the blood sample.

_____ 12. Remove and discard gloves; wash hands.

_____ 13. Ensure that the blood sample is delivered to the proper laboratory for testing.

_____ 14. Document and report the results to the RN or preceptor.

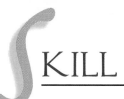# SKILL

Measuring Bleeding Time

Purpose Bleeding time is primarily a screening test for coagulation disorders. A small incision is made in the forearm (Mielke method) or the earlobe (Duke method), and the time it takes for the bleeding to stop is measured and recorded. Because the Mielke method is used more commonly, it is described here. This test may be requested before surgery or in the diagnosis of Willebrand's disease.

The caregiver demonstrates the ability to do the following:

1. Gather the correct supplies.

2. Communicate using a style that reduces the patient's anxiety.

3. Correctly measure the patient's bleeding time.

4. Report the results of the procedure to the RN or preceptor.

Objectives

Filter Paper Circular pieces of absorbent paper used to absorb blood droplets while measuring bleeding time.

Surgicutt A small handheld device containing an extremely sharp lancet that is used to make an incision to measure bleeding time.

Blood pressure cuff • Clean gloves • Alcohol swab • Dry gauze pads • Surgicutt • Watch with a second hand, or stopwatch • Filter paper • Butterfly bandage

Key Terms

Supplies/
Equipment

- It has been established that aspirin and aspirin-containing drugs can cause bleeding or extend bleeding times. Patients should not take aspirin for 7 to 10 days before the test unless otherwise instructed by their doctor. If the patient has taken aspirin and the test is done, it should be noted on the lab requisition.

- Inform the patient that a faint scar can result from the procedure.

- If bleeding has not stopped after 15 minutes, stop the procedure. Apply the dressing and pressure if necessary to stop the bleeding. It is important to document that the procedure was stopped, and the physician should be notified of the results.

Pertinent
Points

Older adults might not be able to recall or might not be aware if they have taken any aspirin-containing medications during the past week. Ask older patients if they regularly take any medications for headaches or pain. Measuring bleeding time requires that the patient sit still for a short period of time. Be sure that the patient is comfortable before beginning the procedure. Adults of all ages would benefit from some diversion, such as a TV or radio program, to hold their attention.

Age-Specific
Considerations

Key Concepts

- If the patient does not bleed, the procedure should be tried on the other arm. If policy permits, an alternate method—such as the Duke method, in which the earlobe is pierced with two incisions—can be used.
- Never do a bleeding time above an IV site.

1. Wash hands.

2. Assemble the equipment.

3. Identify the correct patient.

4. Explain the procedure to the patient.

5. Place the patient's arm in the supine position. It should be firmly supported, with the volar surface exposed.

6. Place the blood pressure cuff on the upper arm.

7. Put on gloves.

8. Clean the area with an alcohol swab. Let air dry, or dry with gauze. (If the site is particularly hairy, it might need to be clipped or shaved. Follow institution preference.)

9. Remove the Surgicutt (or similar product) from package. Twist off the tear-away tab on the side of the Surgicutt. Do not touch the blade slot or push the trigger.

10. Inflate the blood pressure cuff to 40 mm Hg. The test should be started within 60 seconds after the cuff has been inflated.

11. Place the Surgicutt firmly on the forearm approximately 4 inches from the antecubital fossa. The incision should be parallel to the fold of the elbow.

12. Depress the trigger, and watch the second hand or start the stopwatch. Remove the Surgicutt 1 second after pulling the trigger. Continue timing the bleeding.

13. Use the edge of the filter paper to absorb the flow of blood. Place the filter paper close to the incision site without touching the edge of the wound. Disruption of the platelet plug will prolong bleeding time. Blot every 30 seconds until blood no longer stains the filter paper (Figure 5.9). Stop timing.

14. Remove the cuff, gently clean the arm, and apply a butterfly bandage across the incision. Instruct the patient to keep the bandage in place for 24 hours.

15. Dispose of all waste in the proper receptacle.

16. Remove and discard gloves; wash hands.

17. Document and report the results of the procedure, as well as patient tolerance, to the RN or preceptor. A copy of the requisition needs to go to the coagulation department, or the physician need to be notified of the results. Follow institution policy.

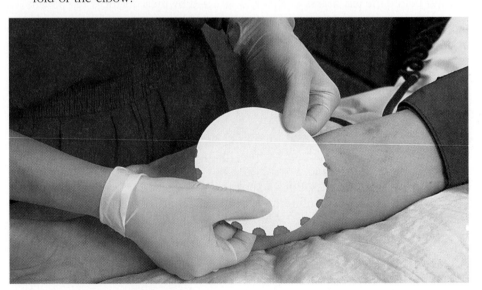

Figure 5.9 Measuring bleeding times.

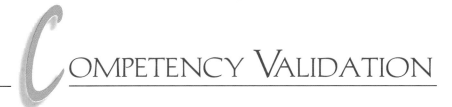

COMPETENCY VALIDATION

Skill: Measuring Bleeding Time

Name _____

Preceptor _____

Date _____

Competency Statement Measures bleeding time while demonstrating correct sterile technique.

Not Competent: _____ 1. Is <u>unable to state reason</u> for task and <u>needs instructions</u> to perform task.

_____ 2. Understands reason for task but <u>needs instructions</u> to perform task.

Competent: _____ 3. Understands reason for task and is able to perform task but <u>needs to increase speed.</u>

_____ 4. Understands reason for task and is able to perform task <u>proficiently.</u>

Performance Criteria

The caregiver demonstrates the ability to do the following:

_____ 1. Wash hands.

_____ 2. Assemble the equipment.

_____ 3. Identify the correct patient.

_____ 4. Explain the procedure to the patient.

_____ 5. Place the patient's arm in the supine position. It should be firmly supported, with the volar surface exposed.

_____ 6. Place the blood pressure cuff on the upper arm.

_____ 7. Put on gloves.

_____ 8. Clean the area with an alcohol swab. Let air dry, or dry with gauze. (If the site is particularly hairy, it may need to be clipped or shaved. Follow institution preference.)

_____ 9. Remove the Surgicutt (or similar product) from package. Twist off the tear-away tab on the side of the Surgicutt. Do not touch the blade slot or push the trigger.

_____ 10. Inflate the blood pressure cuff to 40 mm Hg. The test should be started within 60 seconds after the cuff has been inflated.

_____ 11. Place the Surgicutt firmly on the forearm approximately 4 inches from the antecubital fossa. The incision should be parallel to the fold of the elbow.

_____ 12. Depress the trigger, and watch the second hand or start the stopwatch. Remove the Surgicutt 1 second after pulling the trigger. Continue timing the bleeding.

_____ 13. Use the edge of the filter paper to absorb the flow of blood. Place the filter paper close to the incision site without touching the edge of the wound. Disruption of the platelet plug will prolong bleeding time. Blot every 30 seconds until blood no longer stains the filter paper. Stop timing.

_____ 14. Remove the cuff, gently clean the arm, and apply a butterfly bandage across the incision. Instruct the patient to keep the bandage in place for 24 hours.

_____ 15. Dispose of all waste in the proper receptacle.

_____ 16. Remove and discard gloves; wash hands.

_____ 17. Document and report the results of the procedure, as well as patient tolerance, to the RN or preceptor. A copy of the requisition might need to go to the coagulation department, or the physician might need to be notified of the results. Follow institution policy.

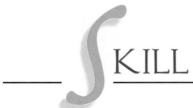

SECTION TWO
IV Therapy

SKILL

Inserting a Heplock

Purpose The insertion of a tube into a patient's vein to provide direct access to the patient's bloodstream is known as IV therapy. A heparin lock, or heplock, is used when the continuous infusion of IV fluids is not necessary. The heplock (or saline lock) is often used for intermittent administration of IV antibiotics or other medications that the physician has ordered to be given at specific times, such as every 6 hours or PRN, such as for pain medications as needed. Another common use for a heplock is with unstable patients who might need emergency medications for a rapid change in condition but who do not require extra fluids.

Objectives

The caregiver demonstrates the ability to do the following:

1. Receive specific instructions from the RN and check the physician's order on the patient's chart.
2. Gather the correct supplies.
3. Communicate using a style that reduces the patient's anxiety.
4. Maintain sterile technique.
5. Use standard precautions.
6. Evaluate and select the most appropriate vein.
7. Select an IV catheter that is appropriate for the size of the patient's veins and the purpose of the IV therapy.
8. Insert the IV catheter, attach the heplock adapter, flush with saline or heparin per institution policy, and correctly apply dressing.
9. Dispose of the needle in a sharps container.
10. Document the procedure correctly in the patient's chart.
11. Report the results of the procedure to the RN or preceptor.

Key Terms

Antecubital Related to the space in the bend of the elbow.

Bevel The slanted edge at the opening of a needle or catheter.

Distal Farthest from the heart.

Gauge The size or measurement of the diameter of a needle or catheter opening (for example, 14, 16, 18, 20, 22, 24). The larger the number, the smaller the diameter of the needle or catheter. Needles are usually sized in odd numbers, catheters in even numbers.

Palpation Examination by touch, such as the examination of a vein by touch to determine its size, elasticity, and location.

Proximal Closest to the heart.

Stylet The needle inside a catheter.

Intermittent injection adapter • 3-cc syringe filled with normal saline or heplock solution, per institution policy • Towel or protective pad • Tourniquet • Clean disposable gloves • Alcohol swabs or povidone-iodine swabs • IV catheter • Sterile 2×2s • Transparent dressing • Tape

- A physician's order is required to start or discontinue a heplock.

- Because this procedure involves inserting a catheter and often medications and fluids directly into the patient's bloodstream, strict sterile technique is required to prevent exposing the patient to a potentially life-threatening infection.

- As with an IV, when selecting a vein for a heplock, choose the distal veins first. For later heplock starts, use the more proximal portions of the vein, thereby working your way up the patient's arms through the course of therapy. This method of site selection prevents irritating fluids from being infused into previously used veins.

Patients of any age might fear being stuck with a needle. Explain the procedure and the therapy in terms that the patient can understand. Be sure to have assistance, as needed, to hold a child or a confused patient to prevent movement during the insertion. Children and geriatric patients sometimes have small or fragile veins, requiring the use of smaller catheters to start the heplock.

*T*he fluid instilled in the lock has long been a controversy in many hospitals. In recent years, many institutions have switched from the anticoagulant heparin to normal saline flushes to maintain patency. Check and follow your institution's policy.

1. Wash hands.
2. Assemble the equipment. Prime the intermittent infusion adapter with normal saline or heplock solution.
3. Identify the correct patient.
4. Explain the procedure to the patient. Determine the patient's preference for site selection if possible.
5. Set up the equipment on the bedside table, within easy reach.
6. Place the towel or protective pad under the patient's arm.
7. Apply the tourniquet to the patient's arm.
8. Palpate the arm, and select a venipuncture site.
9. Remove the tourniquet.
10. Put on gloves.

11. Clean the chosen site with an alcohol or povidone-iodine swab, per institution policy. Use a circular motion, starting at the insertion site and moving slowly outward. Clean for 1 minute. Allow to dry. (Hair at the site may be clipped, if necessary, before cleaning.)
12. Reapply the tourniquet approximately 3 to 4 inches above the selected insertion site.
13. Stabilize the vein with the nondominant hand. Using sterile technique, hold the catheter by the hub. Insert the catheter at a 25- to 45-degree angle, with the bevel pointing up. Firmly pierce the skin.
14. Carefully advance the catheter and stylet into the vein. Observe for blood return.

15. Stabilize the stylet, and advance the catheter into the vein. Do not push the stylet, or needle portion, into the vein.

16. Place a sterile 2×2 beneath the hub of the catheter. Withdraw the stylet most of the way out of the catheter. Put slight pressure over the vein about 1 inch above the insertion site.

17. Remove the tourniquet.

18. Remove the stylet, and place it in a sharps container. Attach the intermittent infusion adapter, and release pressure on the vein.

19. Slowly inject normal saline or heplock solution (Figure 5.10).

20. Observe the site for signs of infiltration: swelling, skin coolness, or blanching.

21. Dress the IV site using a transparent dressing over the insertion site and tape to secure the hub.

22. Label the dressing with the date, the catheter size, and your initials.

23. Remove and discard gloves; wash hands.

24. Document and report the results of the procedure, as well as patient tolerance, to the RN or preceptor.

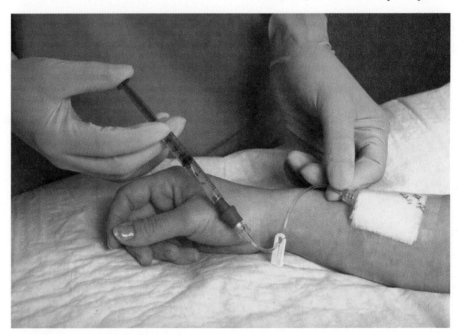

Figure 5.10 Injecting normal saline in a heplock.

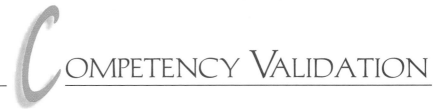
Name _____

Preceptor _____

Date _____

Competency Statement   Inserts a heplock while demonstrating correct sterile technique.

Not Competent: _____ 1. Is <u>unable to state reason</u> for task and <u>needs instructions</u> to perform task.

_____ 2. Understands reason for task but <u>needs instructions</u> to perform task.

Competent: _____ 3. Understands reason for task and is able to perform task but <u>needs to increase speed.</u>

_____ 4. Understands reason for task and is able to perform task <u>proficiently.</u>

Performance Criteria

The caregiver demonstrates the ability to do the following:

_____ 1. Wash hands.

_____ 2. Assemble the equipment. Prime the intermittent infusion adapter with normal saline or heplock solution.

_____ 3. Identify the patient.

_____ 4. Explain the procedure to the patient. Determine the patient's preference for site selection if possible.

_____ 5. Set up the equipment on the bedside table, within easy reach.

_____ 6. Place the towel or protective pad under the patient's arm.

_____ 7. Apply the tourniquet to the patient's arm.

_____ 8. Palpate the arm, and select a venipuncture site.

_____ 9. Remove the tourniquet.

_____ 10. Put on gloves.

_____ 11. Clean the chosen site with an alcohol or povidone-iodine swab, per institution policy. Use a circular motion, starting at the insertion site and moving slowly outward. Clean for 1 minute. Allow to dry. (Hair at the site may be clipped, if necessary, before cleaning.)

_____ 12. Reapply the tourniquet approximately 3 to 4 inches above the selected insertion site.

_____ 13. Stabilize the vein with the nondominant hand. Using sterile technique, hold the catheter by the hub. Insert the catheter at a 25- to 45-degree angle, with the bevel pointing up. Firmly pierce the skin.

_____ 14. Carefully advance the catheter and stylet into the vein. Observe for blood return.

_____ 15. Stabilize the stylet, and advance the catheter into the vein. Do not push the stylet, or needle portion, into the vein.

_____ 16. Place a sterile 2×2 beneath the hub of the catheter. Withdraw the stylet most of the way out of the catheter. Put slight pressure over the vein about 1 inch above the insertion site.

_____ 17. Remove the tourniquet.

_____ 18. Remove the stylet, and place it in a sharps container. Attach the intermittent infusion adapter, and release pressure on the vein.

_____ 19. Slowly inject normal saline or heplock solution.

_____ 20. Observe the site for signs of infiltration: swelling, skin coolness, or blanching.

_____ 21. Dress the IV site using a transparent dressing over the insertion site and tape to secure the hub.

_____ 22. Label the dressing with the date, the catheter size, and your initials.

_____ 23. Remove and discard gloves; wash hands.

_____ 24. Document and report the results of the procedure, as well as patient tolerance, to the RN or preceptor.

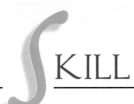

SKILL

Inserting a Butterfly (Winged Infusion Device)

Purpose The insertion of a tube into a patient's vein to supply fluid, salts, glucose, vitamins, or medications is called IV therapy. A butterfly device is usually used for short-term IV therapy, such as infusing chemotherapy IV push, or for difficult blood drawing.

Objectives

The caregiver demonstrates the ability to do the following:

1. Receive specific instructions from the RN and/or check the physician's order on the patient's chart.

2. Identify the type of IV fluid, the size of the bag, and the flow rate ordered.

3. Gather the correct supplies.

4. Communicate using a style that reduces the patient's anxiety.

5. Maintain sterile technique and use standard precautions.

6. Correctly set up the IV bag and tubing.

7. Evaluate and select the most appropriate vein.

8. Select an IV catheter that is appropriate for the size of the patient's veins and the purpose of the IV therapy.

9. Insert the butterfly, attach the tubing, and apply the dressing correctly.

10. Set the IV rate per the physician's order.

11. Document the procedure correctly in the patient's chart.

12. Report the results of the procedure to the RN or preceptor.

Key Terms

Antecubital Related to the space in the bend of the elbow.

Bevel The slanted edge at the opening of a needle or catheter.

Distal Farthest from the heart.

Gauge The size or measurement of the diameter of a needle or catheter opening (for example, 19,21,23,25). The larger the number, the smaller the diameter of the needle or catheter. Needles are usually sized in odd numbers, catheters in even numbers.

Palpation Examination by touch, such as the examination of a vein by touch to determine its size, elasticity, and location.

Proximal Closest to the heart.

Spike To insert an administration set into an IV bag or bottle.

Venipuncture Insertion of a needle through the skin into a peripheral vein to draw blood or insert an IV device.

Supplies/ Equipment

Butterflies of various sizes • Saline-filled syringe • Towel or protective pad • Tourniquet • Clean disposable gloves • Alcohol swabs or povidone-iodine swabs • Appropriate IV bag or bottle and IV tubing • Sterile 2×2s • Transparent dressing • Tape

- A physician's order is required to start, change, maintain, or discontinue IV therapy.
- Because this procedure involves inserting a needle and often medications and fluids directly into the patient's bloodstream, strict sterile technique is required to prevent exposing the patient to a potentially life-threatening infection.
- Due to the inflexibility of the butterfly needle, it is used only when very frequent observation of the site is possible throughout therapy.

Pertinent Points

Patients of any age might fear being stuck with a needle, and the sight of a person coming into the room with an IV pole and other assorted equipment might produce anxiety. Explain the procedure and the therapy in terms that the patient can understand. Be sure to have assistance, as needed, to hold an infant, a small child, or a confused patient to prevent movement during the insertion.

Children and geriatric patients sometimes have small or fragile veins, requiring the use of smaller-gauge butterflies to start the IV. A child's IV must be taped very securely so that it will not become dislodged with activity or during play. A butterfly may be used to start a scalp vein IV in infants.

Age-Specific Considerations

Key Concept

*T*he butterfly should not be used in veins that run over joints unless total immobilization of the joint is possible. Arm boards are frequently used for this purpose.

Steps

1. Wash hands.
2. Assemble the equipment. Prime the butterfly tubing using a saline-filled syringe.
3. Identify the correct patient.
4. Explain the procedure to the patient. Determine the patient's preference for site selection if possible.
5. Set up the equipment on the bedside table, within easy reach.
6. Place the towel or protective pad under the patient's arm.
7. Apply the tourniquet to the patient's arm (Figure 5.11).

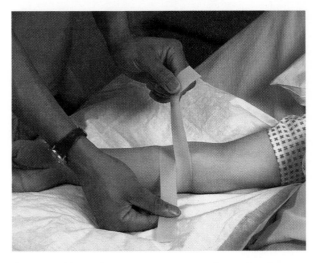 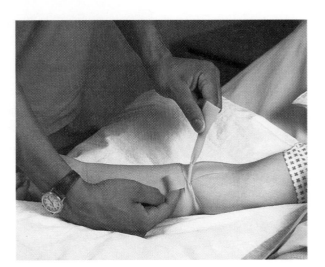

Figure 5.11 Applying a tourniquet to the patient's arm.

8. Palpate the arm, and select an insertion site. The site chosen must allow insertion into a straight length of vein; because the butterfly is inflexible, it could easily go through a vein (Figure 5.12).

9. Remove the tourniquet.

10. Put on gloves.

11. Clean the chosen IV site with an alcohol or povidone-iodine swab, per institution policy. Use a circular motion, starting at the insertion site and moving slowly outward. Clean for 1 minute. Allow to dry. (Hair at the site may be clipped, if necessary, before cleaning.)

12. Reapply the tourniquet approximately 3 to 4 inches above the selected insertion site.

13. Stabilize the vein with the nondominant hand. Grasp the butterfly by folding the wings together with the bevel of the needle up. Firmly pierce the skin, and slide the needle into the vein up to the wings in one smooth movement.

14. Observe for blood return in the butterfly tubing.

15. Remove the tourniquet.

16. Attach the IV tubing.

17. Open the IV fluid to run at a slow rate.

18. Observe the site for signs of infiltration: swelling, skin coolness, or blanching.

19. Dress the IV site using a transparent dressing over the insertion site and tape to secure the hub and IV tubing.

20. Label the dressing with the date, the catheter size, and your initials.

21. Set the IV rate as ordered by the physician.

22. Remove and discard gloves; wash hands.

23. Document and report the results of the procedure, as well as patient tolerance, to the RN or preceptor.

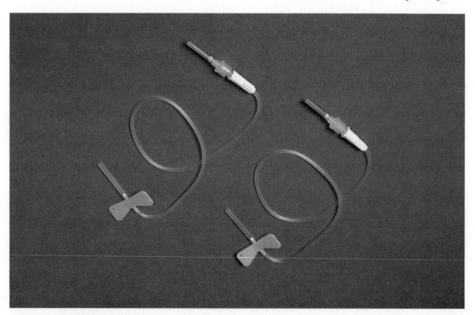

Figure 5.12 Winged or butterfly needle.

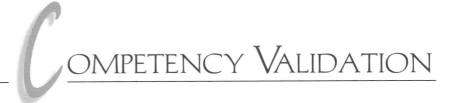

COMPETENCY VALIDATION

Skill: Inserting a Butterfly (Winged Infusion Device)

Name _____

Preceptor _____

Date _____

Competency Statement

Inserts a butterfly (winged infusion device) while demonstrating correct sterile technique.

Not Competent: _____ 1. Is <u>unable to state reason</u> for task and <u>needs instructions</u> to perform task.

_____ 2. Understands reason for task but <u>needs instructions</u> to perform task.

Competent: _____ 3. Understands reason for task and is able to perform task but <u>needs to increase speed.</u>

_____ 4. Understands reason for task and is able to perform task <u>proficiently.</u>

Performance Criteria

The caregiver demonstrates the ability to do the following:

_____ 1. Wash hands.

_____ 2. Assemble the equipment. Prime the butterfly tubing with saline.

_____ 3. Identify the correct patient.

_____ 4. Explain the procedure to the patient. Determine the patient's preference for site selection if possible.

_____ 5. Set up the equipment on the bedside table, within easy reach.

_____ 6. Place the towel or protective pad under the patient's arm.

_____ 7. Apply the tourniquet to the patient's arm.

_____ 8. Palpate the arm, and select an insertion site. The site chosen must allow insertion into a straight length of vein; because the butterfly is inflexible, it could easily go through a vein.

_____ 9. Remove the tourniquet.

_____ 10. Put on gloves.

_____ 11. Clean the chosen IV site with an alcohol or povidone-iodine swab, per institution policy. Use a circular motion, starting at the insertion site and moving slowly outward. Clean for 1 minute. Allow to dry. (Hair at the site may be clipped, if necessary, before cleaning.)

_____ 12. Reapply the tourniquet approximately 3 to 4 inches above the selected insertion site.

_____ 13. Stabilize the vein with the nondominant hand. Grasp the butterfly by folding the wings together with the bevel of the needle up. Firmly pierce the skin, and slide the needle into the vein up to the wings in one smooth movement.

_____ 14. Observe for blood return in the butterfly tubing.

_____ 15. Remove the tourniquet.

_____ 16. Attach the IV tubing.

_____ 17. Open the IV fluid to run at a slow rate.

_____ 18. Observe the site for signs of infiltration: swelling, skin coolness, or blanching.

_____ 19. Dress the IV site using a transparent dressing over the insertion site and tape to secure the hub and IV tubing.

_____ 20. Label the dressing with the date, the catheter size, and your initials.

_____ 21. Set the IV rate as ordered by the physician.

_____ 22. Remove and discard gloves; wash hands.

_____ 23. Document and report the results of the procedure, as well as patient tolerance, to the RN or preceptor.

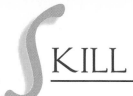

SKILL

Inserting a Peripheral IV in an Adult

Purpose   The insertion of a tube into a patient's vein to provide direct access to the patient's bloodstream is called IV therapy. The IV route may be used to supply fluid when patients are unable to take adequate amounts by mouth, to provide salts needed to maintain electrolyte balance, to provide glucose as fuel for metabolism, to provide water-soluble vitamins and medications, and to establish a lifeline for rapidly needed medications.

Objectives

The caregiver demonstrates the ability to do the following:

1. Receive specific instructions from the RN and check the physician's order on the patient's chart.

2. Identify the type of IV fluid, the size of the bag, and the flow rate ordered.

3. Gather the correct supplies.

4. Communicate using a style that reduces the patient's anxiety.

5. Maintain sterile technique and follow standard precautions.

6. Correctly set up the IV bag and tubing.

7. Evaluate and select the most appropriate vein.

8. Select an IV catheter that is appropriate for the size of the patient's veins and the purpose of the IV therapy.

9. Insert the IV catheter, attach the tubing, and apply the dressing correctly.

10. Dispose of the needle in the sharps container.

11. Set the IV rate per the physician's order.

12. Document the procedure correctly in the patient's chart.

13. Report the results of the procedure to the RN or preceptor.

Key Terms

Antecubital Related to the space in the bend of the elbow.

Bevel The slanted edge at the opening of a needle or catheter.

Distal Farthest from the heart.

Gauge The size or measurement of the diameter of a needle or catheter opening (for example, 14, 16, 18, 20, 22, 24). The larger the number, the smaller the diameter of the needle or catheter. Needles are usually sized in odd numbers, catheters in even numbers.

Palpation Examination by touch, such as the examination of a vein by touch to determine its size, elasticity, and location.

Proximal Closest to the heart.

Spike To insert an administration set into an IV bag or bottle.

Stylet The needle inside a catheter.

Venipuncture Insertion of a needle through the skin into a peripheral vein to draw blood or insert an IV device.

Appropriate IV bag or bottle and IV tubing, primed • Towel or protective pad • Tourniquet • Clean disposable gloves • Alcohol swabs or povidone-iodine swabs • IV catheters of various sizes • Sterile 2×2s • Transparent dressing • Tape

- A physician's order is required to start, change, maintain, or discontinue IV therapy.

- Because this procedure involves inserting a catheter and often medications and fluids directly into the patient's bloodstream, strict sterile technique is required to prevent exposing the patient to a potentially life-threatening infection.

- If the duration of the IV therapy is expected to be long (that is, more than a few hours), several factors must be taken into account when choosing the site. If patients are to be able to feed, bathe, and dress themselves, the caregiver should take into account their ability to move their hand or arm after the IV is placed. Thus the antecubital space and any site over a joint are used only as a last resort for long-term IV therapy.

Patients of any age might fear being stuck with a needle, and the sight of a person coming into the room with an IV pole and other assorted equipment might produce anxiety. Explain the procedure and the therapy in terms that the patient can understand. Be sure to have assistance, as needed, to hold a confused patient to prevent movement during the insertion. Geriatric patients sometimes have small or fragile veins, requiring the use of smaller catheters to start the IV.

- When selecting an initial IV site, use the distal veins first. For subsequent IV starts, choose the more proximal portions of the vein, thereby working your way up the patient's arms through the course of therapy. This method of site selection prevents irritating fluids from being infused into previously used veins.
- Use caution as you advance the catheter into the vein. Do not push the stylet, or needle portion, into the vein.

1. Wash hands.

2. Assemble the equipment. Prime the IV tubing.

3. Identify the correct patient.

4. Explain the procedure to the patient. Determine the patient's preference for site selection if possible.

5. Set up the equipment on the bedside table, within easy reach.

6. Place the towel or protective pad under the patient's arm.

7. Apply the tourniquet to the patient's arm (Figure 5.11).

8. Palpate the arm, and select an IV site.

9. Remove the tourniquet.

10. Put on sterile gloves.

11. Clean the chosen IV site with an alcohol or povidone-iodine swab, per institution policy. Use a circular motion, starting at the insertion site and moving slowly outward (Figure 5.13a). Clean for 1 minute. Allow to dry. (Hair at the site may be clipped, if necessary, before cleaning.)

12. Reapply the tourniquet approximately 3 to 4 inches above the selected insertion site.

13. Stabilize the vein with the non-dominant hand (Figure 5.13b). Using sterile technique, hold the catheter by the hub. Insert the catheter at a 25- to 45-degree angle, with the bevel pointing up. Firmly pierce the skin (Figure 5.13c).

14. Carefully advance the catheter and stylet into the vein (Figure 5.13d). Observe for blood return.

15. Stabilize the stylet, and advance the catheter into the vein. Do not push the stylet, or needle portion, into the vein.

16. Place a sterile 2×2 beneath the hub of the catheter. Withdraw the stylet most of the way out of the catheter. Put slight pressure over the vein about 1 inch above the insertion site.

17. Remove the tourniquet.

18. Remove the stylet, and place it in a sharps container. Attach the IV tubing, and release pressure on the vein (Figure 5.13e).

19. Open the IV fluid to run at a slow rate.

20. Observe the site for signs of infiltration: swelling, skin coolness, or blanching.

21. Dress the IV site using a transparent dressing over the insertion site and tape to secure the hub and IV tubing (Figure 5.13f).

22. Label the dressing with the date, the catheter size, and your initials.

23. Set the IV rate as ordered by the physician.

24. Remove and discard gloves; wash hands.

25. Document and report the results of the procedure, as well as patient tolerance, to the RN or preceptor.

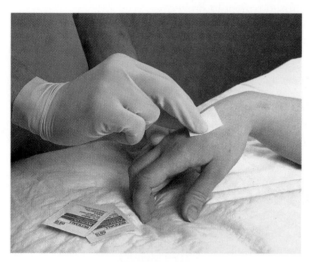

a

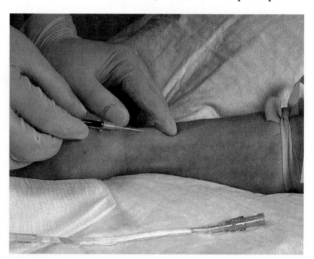

b

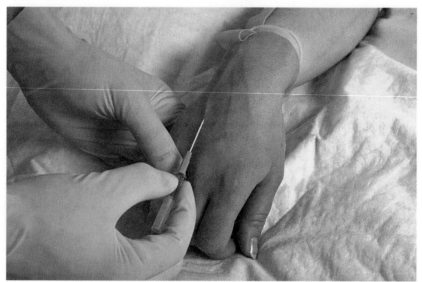

c

Figure 5.13 Inserting a peripheral IV in an adult.

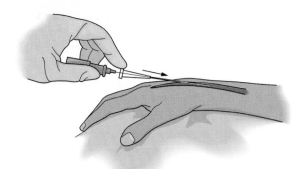

d

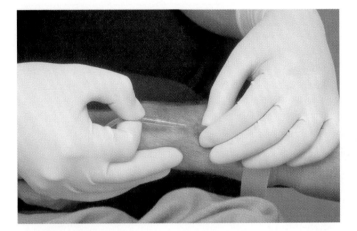

e

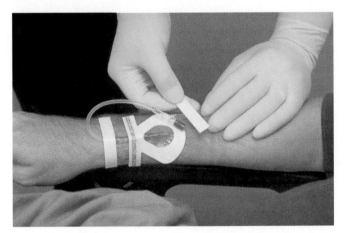

f

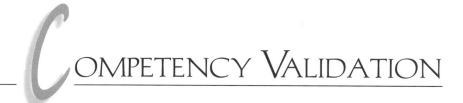

COMPETENCY VALIDATION

Skill: Inserting a Peripheral IV in an Adult

Name _____

Preceptor _____

Date _____

Competency Statement   Inserts a peripheral IV in an adult while demonstrating correct sterile technique.

Not Competent: _____   1. Is <u>unable to state reason</u> for task and <u>needs instructions</u> to perform task.

_____   2. Understands reason for task but <u>needs instructions</u> to perform task.

Competent: _____   3. Understands reason for task and is able to perform task but <u>needs to increase speed.</u>

_____   4. Understands reason for task and is able to perform task <u>proficiently.</u>

Performance Criteria

The caregiver demonstrates the ability to do the following:

_____   1. Wash hands.

_____   2. Assemble the equipment. Prime the IV tubing.

_____   3. Identify the correct patient.

_____   4. Explain the procedure to the patient. Determine the patient's preference for site selection if possible.

_____   5. Set up the equipment on the bedside table, within easy reach.

_____   6. Place the towel or protective pad under the patient's arm.

_____   7. Apply the tourniquet to the patient's arm.

_____   8. Palpate the arm, and select an IV site.

_____   9. Remove the tourniquet.

_____ 10. Put on sterile gloves.

_____ 11. Clean the chosen IV site with an alcohol or povidone-iodine swab, per institution policy. Use a circular motion, starting at the insertion site and moving slowly outward. Clean for one minute. Allow to dry. (Hair at the site may be clipped, if necessary, before cleaning.)

_____ 12. Reapply the tourniquet approximately 3 to 4 inches above the selected insertion site.

_____ 13. Stabilize the vein with the nondominant hand. Using sterile technique, hold the catheter by the hub. Insert the catheter at a 25- to 45-degree angle, with the bevel pointing up. Firmly pierce the skin.

_____ 14. Carefully advance the catheter and stylet into the vein. Observe for blood return.

_____ 15. Stabilize the stylet, and advance the catheter into the vein. Do not push the stylet, or needle portion, into the vein.

_____ 16. Place a sterile 2×2 beneath the hub of the catheter. Withdraw the stylet most of the way out of the catheter. Put slight pressure over the vein about 1 inch above the insertion site.

_____ 17. Remove the tourniquet.

_____ 18. Remove the stylet, and place it in a sharps container. Attach the IV tubing, and release pressure on the vein.

_____ 19. Open the IV fluid to run at a slow rate.

_____ 20. Observe the site for signs of infiltration: swelling, skin coolness, or blanching.

_____ 21. Dress the IV site using a transparent dressing over the insertion site and tape to secure the hub and IV tubing.

_____ 22. Label the dressing with the date, the catheter size, and your initials.

_____ 23. Set the IV rate as ordered by the physician.

_____ 24. Remove and discard gloves; wash hands.

_____ 25. Document and report the results of the procedure, as well as patient tolerance, to the RN or preceptor.

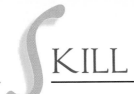

SKILL

Inserting a Peripheral IV in a Child

Purpose   The insertion of a tube into a patient's vein to provide direct access to the patient's bloodstream is called IV therapy. Pediatric patients become dehydrated more easily than adults. IV fluids are often used to replace fluids and electrolytes lost through fever, vomiting, or diarrhea.

The caregiver demonstrates the ability to do the following:

Objectives

1. Receive specific instructions from the RN and check the physician's order on the patient's chart.
2. Identify the type of IV fluid, the size of the bag, and the flow rate ordered.
3. Gather the correct supplies.
4. Communicate using a style that reduces the patient's anxiety.
5. Maintain sterile technique and follow standard precautions.
6. Correctly set up the IV bag and tubing.
7. Evaluate and select the most appropriate vein.
8. Select an IV catheter that is appropriate for the size of the patient's veins and the purpose of the IV therapy.
9. Ensure adequate assistance to hold the child securely.
10. Insert the IV catheter, attach the tubing, and apply the dressing correctly.
11. Dispose of the needle in the sharps container.
12. Set the IV rate per the physician's order.
13. Document the procedure correctly in the patient's chart.
14. Report the results of the procedure to the RN or preceptor.

Key Terms

Antecubital Related to the space in the bend of the elbow.

Bevel The slanted edge at the opening of a needle or catheter.

Distal Farthest from the heart.

Gauge The size or measurement of the diameter of a needle or catheter opening (for example, 14, 16, 18, 20, 22, 24). The larger the number, the smaller the diameter of the needle or catheter. Needles are usually sized in odd numbers, catheters in even numbers.

Palpation Examination by touch, such as the examination of a vein by touch to determine its size, elasticity, and location.

Proximal Closest to the heart.

Spike To insert an administration set into an IV bag or bottle.

Stylet The needle inside a catheter.

Venipuncture Insertion of a needle through the skin into a peripheral vein to draw blood or insert an IV device.

Appropriate IV bag or bottle and IV tubing with volume-limiting reservoir (such as Buretrol), primed • Towel or protective pad • Pediatric tourniquet • Arm board • Tape • Sterile disposable gloves • Alcohol swabs • Small IV catheters of various sizes • Sterile 2x2s • Transparent dressing

Pertinent
Points

• A physician's order is required to start, change, maintain, or discontinue IV therapy.

• Because this procedure involves inserting a catheter and often medications and fluids directly into the patient's bloodstream, strict sterile technique is required to prevent exposing the patient to a potentially life-threatening infection.

• The most frequently used sites for pediatric patients are the dorsum of the hand, the dorsum of the foot, and the scalp veins (Figure 5.14).

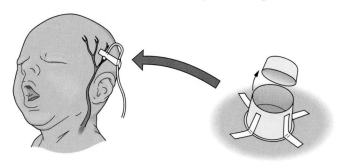

Venipuncture of scalp vein

Paper cup taped over venipuncture site for protection. A clear plastic cup may also be used.

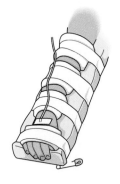 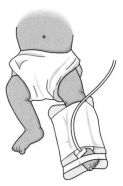

Restraint of arm when
hand is site of infusion

Infant's leg taped to sand-
bag for immobilization

Figure 5.14 IV sites on infant scalp, arm, and leg.

Age-Specific
Considerations

Children often fear needles. Explain the procedure and the therapy in terms that the patient can understand. Be sure to have assistance, as needed, to hold the infant or child to prevent movement during the insertion. Children often have small or fragile veins, requiring the use of small catheters (22 or 24 gauge) to start an IV. Do not tell pediatric patients that the procedure will not hurt. Be truthful, but explain that the needle will hurt only for a short time. The IV must be taped very securely so that it will not become dislodged with activity or during play.

Key Concept

*U*se caution when advancing the catheter into the vein. Do not push the stylet, or needle portion, into the vein.

1. Wash hands.

2. Assemble the equipment. Prime the IV tubing, and fill the volume-limiting reservoir.

3. Identify the correct patient.

4. Explain the procedure to the patient. Use words that the child can understand.

5. Set up the equipment on the bedside table, within easy reach.

6. Place the towel or protective pad under the patient's arm.

7. Apply the tourniquet to the patient's arm.

8. Palpate the arm and select an IV site.

9. Remove the tourniquet.

10. Secure the arm to the arm board with tape, leaving the insertion site uncovered. Have an assistant hold the limb securely without cutting off circulation.

11. Put on gloves.

12. Clean the chosen IV site with an alcohol swab. Use a circular motion, starting at the insertion site and moving slowly outward. Clean for 1 minute. Allow to dry.

13. Reapply the tourniquet approximately 2 to 3 inches above the selected insertion site.

14. Stabilize the vein with the non-dominant hand. Using sterile technique, hold the catheter by the hub. Insert the catheter at a 25- to 35-degree angle, with the bevel pointing up. Firmly pierce the skin.

15. Carefully advance the catheter and stylet into the vein. Observe for blood return.

16. Stabilize the stylet, and advance the catheter into the vein. Do not push the stylet, or needle portion, into the vein.

17. Place a sterile 2×2 beneath the hub of the catheter. Withdraw the stylet most of the way out of the catheter. Put slight pressure over the vein about 1 inch above the insertion site.

18. Remove the tourniquet.

19. Remove the stylet, and place it in the sharps container. Attach the IV tubing, and release the pressure on the vein.

20. Open the IV fluid to run at a slow rate.

21. Observe the site for signs of infiltration: swelling, skin coolness, or blanching.

22. Dress the IV site using a transparent dressing over the insertion site and tape to secure the hub and IV tubing. The arm board may be removed or readjusted as necessary to secure the IV and prevent its accidental removal.

23. Label the dressing with the date, the catheter size, and your initials.

24. Remove and discard gloves; wash hands.

25. Set the IV rate as ordered by the physician.

26. Document and report the results of the procedure, as well as patient tolerance, to the RN or preceptor.

Note: IVs may also be inserted into scalp veins in infants with a physician's order. This procedure requires specialized training and preceptoring by a practitioner experienced in scalp vein IV placement.

Steps

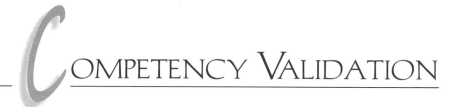

COMPETENCY VALIDATION

Skill: Inserting a Peripheral IV in a Child

Name _____

Preceptor _____

Date _____

Competency Statement Inserts a peripheral IV in a child while demonstrating correct sterile technique.

Not Competent: _____ 1. Is <u>unable to state reason</u> for task and <u>needs instructions</u> to perform task.

_____ 2. Understands reason for task but <u>needs instructions</u> to perform task.

Competent: _____ 3. Understands reason for task and is able to perform task but <u>needs to increase speed.</u>

_____ 4. Understands reason for task and is able to perform task <u>proficiently.</u>

Performance Criteria

The caregiver demonstrates the ability to do the following:

_____ 1. Wash hands.

_____ 2. Assemble the equipment. Prime the IV tubing, and fill the volume-limiting reservoir.

_____ 3. Identify the correct patient.

_____ 4. Explain the procedure to the patient. Use words that the child can understand.

_____ 5. Set up the equipment on the bedside table, within easy reach.

_____ 6. Place the towel or protective pad under the patient's arm.

_____ 7. Apply the tourniquet to the patient's arm.

_____ 8. Palpate the arm, and select an IV site.

_____ 9. Remove the tourniquet.

_____ 10. Secure the arm to the arm board with tape, leaving the insertion site uncovered. Have an assistant hold the limb securely without cutting off circulation.

_____ 11. Put on gloves.

_____ 12. Clean the chosen IV site with an alcohol swab. Use a circular motion, starting at the insertion site and moving slowly outward. Clean for 1 minute. Allow to dry.

_____ 13. Reapply the tourniquet approximately 2 to 3 inches above the selected insertion site.

_____ 14. Stabilize the vein with the nondominant hand. Using sterile technique, hold the catheter by the hub. Insert the catheter at a 25- to 35-degree angle, with the bevel pointing up. Firmly pierce the skin.

_____ 15. Carefully advance the catheter and stylet into the vein. Observe for blood return.

_____ 16. Stabilize the stylet, and advance the catheter into the vein. Do not push the stylet, or needle portion, into the vein.

_____ 17. Place a sterile 2×2 beneath the hub of the catheter. Withdraw the stylet most of the way out of the catheter. Put slight pressure over the vein about 1 inch above the insertion site.

_____ 18. Remove the tourniquet.

_____ 19. Remove the stylet, and place it in the sharps container. Attach the IV tubing, and release the pressure on the vein.

_____ 20. Open the IV fluid to run at a slow rate.

_____ 21. Observe the site for signs of infiltration: swelling, skin coolness, or blanching.

_____ 22. Dress the IV site using a transparent dressing over the insertion site and tape to secure the hub and IV tubing. The arm board may be removed or readjusted as necessary to secure the IV and prevent its accidental removal.

_____ 23. Label the dressing with the date, the catheter size, and your initials.

_____ 24. Remove and discard gloves; wash hands.

_____ 25. Set the IV rate as ordered by the physician.

_____ 26. Document and report the results of the procedure, as well as patient tolerance, to the RN or preceptor.

Recognizing Problems in IV Therapy

Complications of IV therapy can be either local or systemic. Local complications tend to be less serious or life-threatening in nature than systemic ones. The key to managing local complications is frequent observation and assessment of the IV site, prevention by strict asepsis in starting and maintaining the IV, and teaching the patient to observe for early signs of problems.

Infiltration

When the IV device, needle or catheter, comes out of the vein, IV fluids and medications can flow into the surrounding tissues. This is referred to as infiltration. When a particularly irritating drug—a vesicant—infiltrates, it is called extravasation.

The signs and symptoms of infiltration are coolness, blanching or paleness of the adjacent skin, swelling or tautness around the insertion site, discomfort, dependent edema, absence of a blood return, and slowing of the IV rate when infusing by gravity (Figure 5.15).

Techniques for prevention begin with appropriate site selection, selection of veins that avoid joints or can be readily stabilized, proper dressing techniques, and avoidance of high-pressure infusion pumps. Early recognition of infiltration requires frequent monitoring of the IV site and teaching the patient to report signs of infiltration immediately.

Treatment consists of stopping the infusion, discontinuing the IV, elevating the extremity, and using warm compresses to aid in the reabsorption of the fluid.

Streaking or Phlebitis

Phlebitis or streaking is an inflammation of the interior surface of a vein (Figure 5.16). It is a common complication of IV therapy. There are two types of phlebitis: mechanical and chemical. Mechanical phlebitis is caused when the needle or catheter traumatizes the vein wall. This usually happens when the IV device is not adequately secured to the patient's skin. Chemical phlebitis results when irritating fluids or medications damage the endothelial cells of the vein wall (Figure 5.17).

The signs and symptoms of phlebitis are redness, warmness to the touch, local swelling, and palpable venous cord. The formation of phlebitis is affected by insertion techniques, vein condition, the type and pH of medications infused, and the rate and dilution of infusates, the fluids being infused.

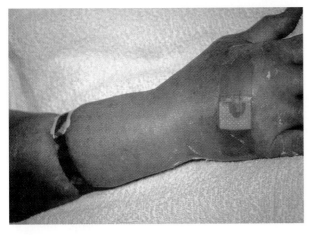

Figure 5.15 Infiltration. (© Johnson & Johnson Medical, Inc. 1997. Used by permission of the copyright owner.)

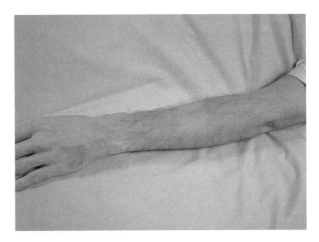

Figure 5.16 Phlebitis. (© Johnson & Johnson Medical, Inc. 1997. Used by permission of the copyright owner.)

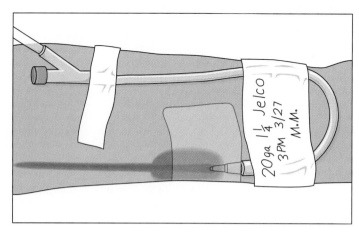

Figure 5.17 Streaking. (© Johnson & Johnson Medical, Inc. 1997. Used by permission of the copyright owner.)

Prevention techniques include using large veins for irritating medications, choosing the smallest IV needle or catheter appropriate for the therapy, rotating the site every 72 hours, stabilizing the IV device, infusing medications slowly and diluting irritating medications, using an in-line filter, and practicing strict aseptic technique when starting and maintaining the IV.

Treatment of phlebitis consists of stopping the IV, removing the IV needle or catheter, and applying warm compresses for comfort. Subsequent IV starts should always be proximal to the previous site of phlebitis.

Ecchymosis or Hematoma

The formation of an ecchymosis, a hematoma, or bruise, at the venipuncture site is usually related to caregiver technique. Bruising can be caused by nicking the vein during an unsuccessful venipuncture attempt or failing to apply pressure over the venipuncture site after the blood draw or after discontinuing an IV device (Figure 5.18).

Prevention includes proper device insertion and the application of pressure over the site after removal of the device.

The signs and symptoms of a hematoma are a darkening or discoloration under the skin at the venipuncture site, swelling at the site, tenderness, and discomfort.

Hematomas can be prevented with the appropriate use of pressure over an IV site after discontinuing the IV device, pressure after blood draws, and care to prevent pushing the needle through the vein during venipuncture.

If the patient develops a hematoma, stop the venipuncture attempt at once, and put pressure over the developing hematoma. Have the patient elevate the extremity to maximize venous return. Careful observation of the venipuncture site when the vein is being pierced will allow the caregiver to discover a hematoma formation early and prevent the further extension of the hematoma. The discoloration will gradually fade, and the blood will be reabsorbed over a period of days to weeks.

IV-Related Infection

Needle or catheter contamination is the most frequent cause of IV-related infection. This is a localized infection at the site of the IV insertion (Figure 5.19).

The signs and symptoms of IV-related infection include redness, swelling, and exudate at the IV insertion site, increased temperature, and elevated white blood cell counts.

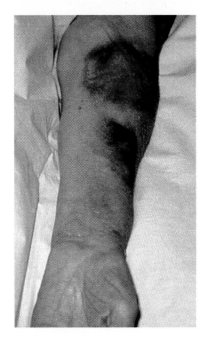 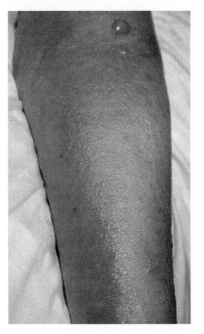 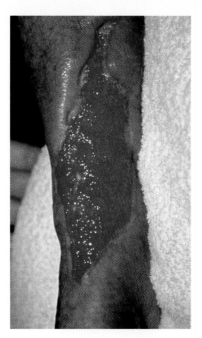

Figure 5.18 Hematoma. (© Johnson & Johnson Medical, Inc. 1997. Used by permission of the copyright owner.)

Figure 5.19 Infection. (© Johnson & Johnson Medical, Inc. 1997. Used by permission of the copyright owner.)

Figure 5.20 Tissue sloughing. (© Johnson & Johnson Medical, Inc. 1997. Used by permission of the copyright owner.)

Local infections are preventable by maintaining strict aseptic technique during insertion, changing the IV site and tubing at CDC-recommended intervals, and careful maintenance of the IV site and dressing during therapy.

If localized infection is suspected, remove the dressing from the IV site. If the symptoms of infection exist, remove the IV device and culture the catheter tip and any purulent drainage from around the site. Notify the patient's physician at once, and send the specimens to the lab for culture as ordered by the physician.

Systemic Complications

The most common systemic complication of peripheral IV therapy is septicemia, which is an invasion of the blood by microorganisms.

The signs and symptoms of septicemia are chills, fever, and malaise. This is a life-threatening problem and if suspected must be reported to the physician immediately. Prompt treatment greatly increases the patient's chance for recovery.

Prevention includes good handwashing and strict aseptic technique during line insertion and maintenance. Filtration of infusate (with a 0.2-micron bacterial-retentive filter) also helps prevent septicemia.

Treatment depends on the results of the culture and must be ordered by the physician on a case-specific basis.

Tissue Sloughing

Tissue sloughing is a serious complication of IV therapy. When sloughing occurs, necrotic tissue forms or separates from viable or healthy tissue (Figure 5.20).

The signs and symptoms include tissue necrosis.

Prevention includes appropriate selection of the site and device, proper stabilization of the device, and frequent checks for signs of infiltration. This is particularly important when irritating solutions or drugs, such as those used to treat cancer (chemotherapy agents), are being administered.

CHAPTER 6
ADVANCED CARDIAC CARE SKILLS

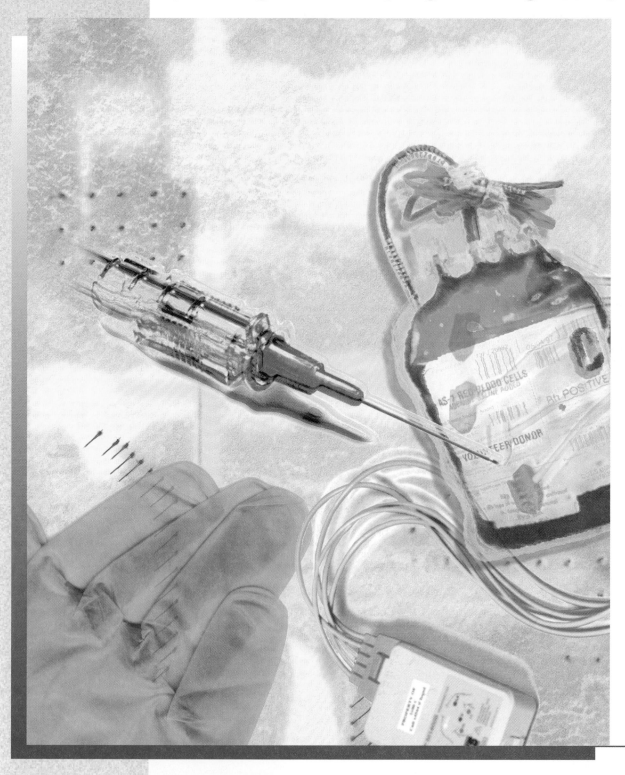

*M*ore and more, nurses and nursing support staff are being asked to perform skills for a growing population of patients with cardiovascular disease. Advanced cardiac skills are becoming necessary tools for caregivers in a variety of settings, from the acute care hospital to the home care environment.

This chapter includes information on the basic anatomy and physiology of the heart. In addition, it prepares caregivers to perform the following skills:

ECG Monitoring and Arrhythmia Recognition

Basic anatomy and physiology of the heart

Relating waveforms on ECG to heart action

Recognizing life-threatening arrhythmias

Setting up continuous three- or five-lead cardiac monitoring and telemetry

Recognizing ECG rhythms that require RN notification or intervention

Advanced Cardiac Care Skills

Performing twelve-lead ECG monitoring

Caring for the patient with an arterial line

Palpating dorsalis pedis and posterior tibial pulses

Removing a PTCA femoral sheath

Performing a postcardiac catheterization check

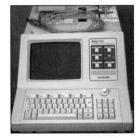
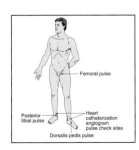
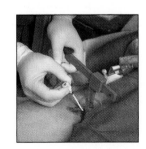

S E C T I O N   O N E
ECG Monitoring and Arrhythmia Recognition

Basic Anatomy and Physiology of the Heart

The heart is a pump that propels oxygen-rich blood to all parts of the body. The human heart has been masterfully designed to respond quickly and efficiently to our physical needs.

This section prepares caregivers to do the following:

1. Describe the basic anatomy and physiology of the heart.

2. Acquire a basic understanding of the conduction system.

3. Relate waveforms on an electrocardiogram to heart action.

Key Terms

Arrhythmia A variation from the normal sinus rhythm.

Atrial Pertaining to an atrium.

Atrium One of two upper chambers of the heart. (Plural is *atria*).

Atrioventricular (AV) Node An area of cardiac muscle fibers lying on the posterior floor of the right atrium that conducts impulses from the atria to the bundle of His. It can also act as a pacemaker of the heart.

Conduction System The cardiac muscle fibers that normally conduct impulses rapidly through the heart to cause depolarization and then contraction to occur. They include the SA node, the AV node, the bundle of His, the right and left bundle branches, and the Purkinje fibers.

Depolarization The spread of an impulse through a chamber of the heart (atrium or ventricle).

Intercostal Space Space between two ribs.

Lead A wire attached to an electrode on the patient's skin that connects in the ECG machine, the bedside monitor, or the telemetry device and transmits electrical information to the monitor or recorder.

Myocardial Infarction A condition in which an area of the heart is deprived of oxygen and the cells die.

Myocardium The middle layer of heart muscle.

Pacemaker (pacer) The site in the heart that initiates the impulses that are spread throughout the cardiac tissue and cause contraction to occur. Normally, the pacemaker of the heart is the SA node, which is located in the right atrium.

Pacemaker Cells A specialized group of cells able to initiate impulses that set the rate of the heartbeat and spread to other areas of the heart.

Precordial Pertaining to an area of the chest over the heart and over the lower portion of the sternum.

Repolarization The recovery period of a chamber of the heart after it has contracted.

Ventricles One of two lower chambers of the heart.

Ventricular Pertaining to a ventricle.

The heart functions to pump blood to the lungs and to the rest of the body. It supplies oxygen- and nutrient-rich blood throughout the body through the circulatory system. The heart consists of four chambers. The two upper chambers are the right and left atriums. The two lower chambers are the right and left ventricles. The right atrium receives blood from the superior vena cava and the inferior vena cava. It contracts to supply the right ventricle with blood, which passes through the tricuspid valve. The right ventricle contracts to move unoxygenated blood along through the pulmonic valve and the pulmonary arteries to the lungs, where the blood receives oxygen. The oxygenated blood then travels back through the pulmonic veins to the left atrium and through the mitral valve to the left ventricle. The left ventricle is responsible for pumping the blood through the aortic valve and aorta to the rest of the body. During ventricular relaxation, blood is supplied to the coronary arteries, which supply oxygenated blood and nutrients to the heart muscle itself (Figure 6.1).

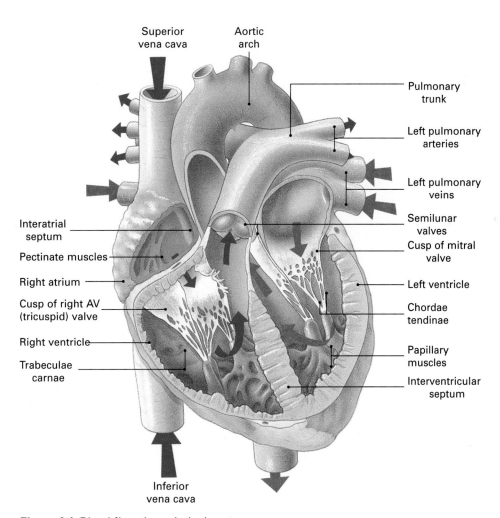

Figure 6.1 Blood flow through the heart.

The coronary circulation consists of two main branches: the left and right coronary arteries. The left main coronary artery divides into the left anterior descending artery (LAD) and the left circumflex artery (LCA) with many additional smaller branches. The LAD supplies blood to the anterior wall of the left ventricle, most of the intraventricular septum, and the bundle branches of the electrical system. The circumflex artery supplies blood to the left atrium, a portion of the lateral wall of the left ventricle, the posterior wall of the left ventricle in some people, and in a small percentage of people the sinoatrial (SA) node and the atrioventricular (AV) node. The right coronary artery (RCA) supplies blood to the right atrium, the right ventricle, and, in the majority of hearts, the SA node and AV node (Figure 6.2).

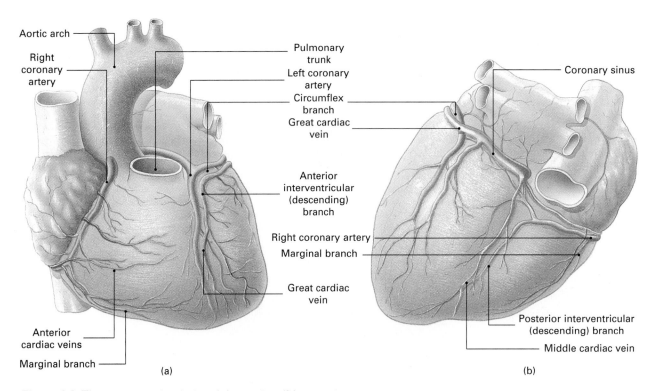

Figure 6.2 The coronary circulation; (**a**) anterior; (**b**) posterior.

The Conductive System

In a normally functioning heart, the SA node acts as the pacemaker of the heart, initiating electrical impulses and spreading the impulse down through the rest of the conduction system, causing depolarization of the muscle cells and, ultimately, contraction of the atria and ventricles. The electrical impulse travels from the SA node through the internodal pathways to the AV node. The AV node delays the impulses from the atria for a short time, allowing for atrial emptying. The impulse then travels through the bundle of His to the right and left bundle branches and, finally, to the Purkinje fibers, which spread throughout the ventricles (Figure 6.3).

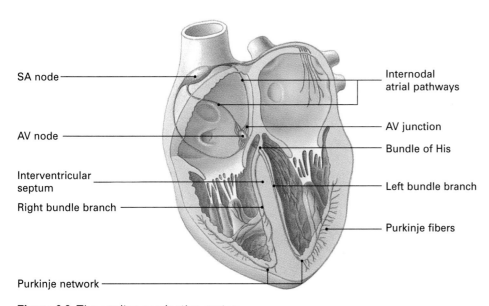

SA node

Internodal atrial pathways

AV node

AV junction

Bundle of His

Interventricular septum

Left bundle branch

Right bundle branch

Purkinje fibers

Purkinje network

Figure 6.3 The cardiac conductive system.

The Electrocardiogram

The terms *ECG* and *EKG* both refer to an electrocardiogram. *EKG* comes from the German spelling (*elektrokardiogram*); and *ECG* reflects the English spelling (*electrocardiogram*). Throughout this text, we will use the term *ECG*.

The first electrocardiogram was reported by Willem Einthoven in the early 1900's. He placed leads on the arms and legs of his subject and measured the electrical activity of the heart with a galvanometer.

ECG monitoring may be done in twelve different leads. Leads I, II, and III are known as bipolar limb leads. Bipolar means that two electrodes, a negative and a positive attached to two extremities, are used to permit a view of the electrical activity from a frontal plane (Figure 6.4). To eliminate electrical interference, a third lead, or ground lead, is commonly used. The three leads aVR, aVL, and aVF are unipolar leads. They look at the heart in a horizontal plane. A unipolar lead is made by attaching a positive electrode on the skin and connecting it with a zero reference point that is made by the machine as it internally connects the extremity electrodes. The aug-

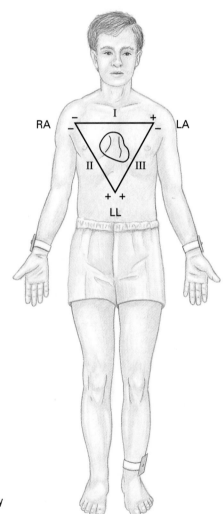

Figure 6.4 Einthoven's triangle as formed by Leads I, II, and III.

mented leads are made by attaching a positive electrode to one of the three extremity leads (the left arm, the right arm, or the left leg). The chest leads (V₁ through V₆) are also unipolar leads. They are known as the precordial leads. Electrodes are placed across the chest in each of the six specified precordial locations.

Electrical Axis or Vector

All of the electrical forces in the heart can be combined into a single vector, or force, that has both magnitude and direction. This vector is usually represented by an arrow. The main vector in a normal heart is downward to the left foot because this is the direction of the normal electrical pathway. If the wave of electrical activity flows toward a positive lead, the pattern will be upright, or positive. If the wave of electrical activity flows away from the positive lead, the pattern will be negative, or inverted. If the wave of electricity flows perpendicular to the positive electrode, the pattern will be isoelectric (Figure 6.5).

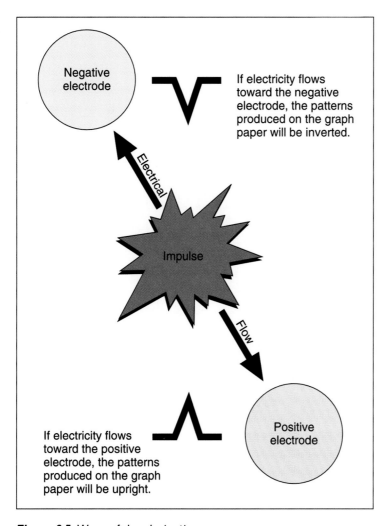

Figure 6.5 Wave of depolorization.

Components of the ECG

An ECG consists of several components. The P wave is small, rounded, and upright. It represents atrial contraction. It is normally the first movement away from the isoelectric line, or baseline, of the ECG. The Q wave is the first negative deflection following a P wave. The R wave is the first positive deflection in the QRS complex following a P wave. The S wave is the first negative complex following the R wave. The S wave normally returns to the isoelectric line before the next wave is seen. The T wave is the next rounded upright wave, and it represents ventricular repolarization (relaxation). The QRS complex represents ventricular depolarization (contraction). The QRS interval is normally 0.06 to 0.11 seconds. The ST segment begins at the end of the QRS and ends at the beginning of the T wave. The PR interval shown in Figure 6.6 represents the time from atrial contraction to the onset of ventricular contraction. The PR interval is measured from the beginning of the P wave to the beginning of the QRS complex. The normal duration of this interval is 0.12 to 0.20 seconds.

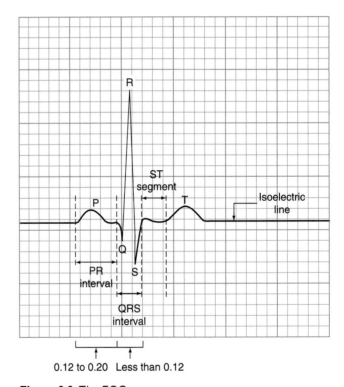

Figure 6.6 The ECG.

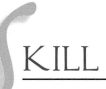

SKILL

Setting Up Continuous Three- or Five-Lead Cardiac Monitoring and Telemetry

Purpose Continuous cardiac monitoring and telemetry are useful diagnostic tools for patients who have had cardiac abnormalities or might be at risk for them. Continuous cardiac monitoring can be performed with a three- or a five-lead setup. The patient is connected to a hardwire monitor with a display at a central monitoring station. Telemetry units, on the other hand, are portable. Their lead wires are connected to a unit that the patient wears in a pocket or a pouch. They offer the advantage of allowing the patient to ambulate without wires connected to a hardwire unit.

The caregiver demonstrates the ability to do the following:

Objectives

1. Gather the correct supplies.
2. Communicate using a style that reduces the patient's anxiety.
3. Set up five-lead hardwire monitoring.
4. Set up three- or five-lead telemetry monitoring.
5. Determine heart rate and regularity.
6. Describe the process of obtaining an ECG.
7. Report the results of the procedure to the RN or preceptor.

Key Terms

Augmented Made larger; increased.

Bigeminy The state of having an ectopic beat that occurs every other beat.

Caliper A tool used to assist in measuring heart rate and rhythm on an ECG strip.

Couplets Two abnormal beats that occur in a row.

Ectopic Situated somewhere other than the normal place.

Ectopy Abnormal beats.

Electrode Gel A gelatinous substance that is used with the ECG electrodes to transmit a good-quality signal to the ECG monitor.

Hardwire Monitoring A monitoring system by which the patient is physically connected to a monitoring device that displays the ECG rhythm at the bedside.

Isoelectric Line The flat area of an ECG where no electrical impulse is detected. Also called baseline.

Multifocal Pertaining to two or more ectopic beats that look different from one another.

Premature Beat A cardiac contraction that occurs before the next normal beat is expected.

Rhythm Strip A long (6 to 12 second) ECG recording of one or more leads during cardiac monitoring.

Stylus The needlelike instrument that writes the heart rhythm onto ECG paper.

Telemetry A system in which the patient is attached to ECG leads and a portable transmitter, which sends radio signals to a central monitor, where the patient's ECG can be viewed.

Unifocal Pertaining to two or more ectopic beats that look alike.

Soap and water • Clippers or scissors to remove hair (if needed) • Pregelled electrodes • Five-lead hardwire monitoring system or three- or five-lead telemetry monitoring system • Carrying pouch or holder for telemetry monitoring unit

Monitoring Methods

Hardwire monitoring usually uses a five-lead system. One end of the leads attaches to a monitor in the patient's room. Lead wires then connect to adhesive electrodes placed on the skin. Five-lead systems offer selection options so that the observer is able to monitor in more than one lead without changing the electrode setup on the chest. Typically, the white lead is on the right arm, the black lead is on the left arm, the green lead (which represents the right foot) is on the right lower abdomen just above the iliac crest, the red lead (representing the left foot) is on the left lower abdomen just above the iliac crest, and the brown lead is in the fourth intercostal space to the right of the sternum (the V_1 position).

A telemetry system uses a portable receiver that transmits ECG data to a central monitoring station. With this system, the patient is able to move about without being confined by wires attached to a monitor in the room. The chest leads connect to a small box that is usually carried in a pouch that the patient wears around the neck or waist.

Five-lead telemetry systems (Figure 6.7) can monitor patients simultaneously in two leads, depending on the monitoring system used (Figures 6.8 and 6.9). Lead MCL_1, the modified chest lead, is a bipolar lead that simulates lead V_1 of the twelve-

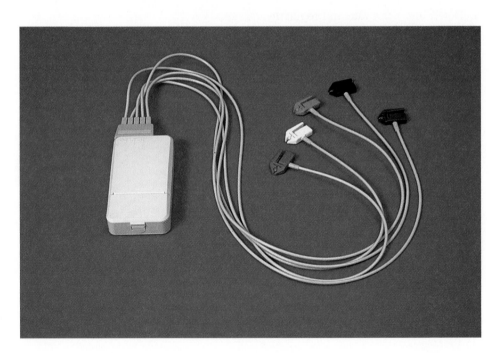

Figure 6.7 Telemetry and leads.

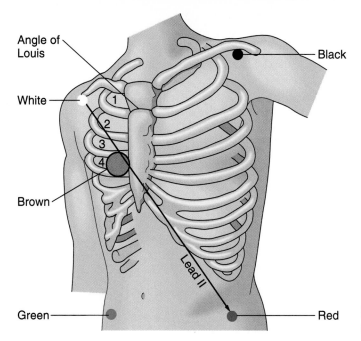

Figure 6.8 Telemetry setup using a five-lead cable (Lead II).

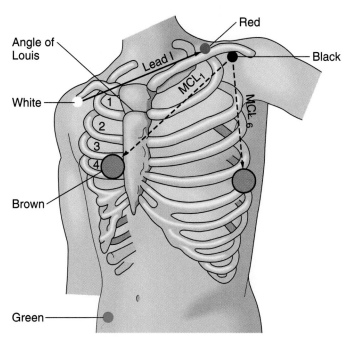

Figure 6.9 Telemetry setup using a five-lead cable (Lead I, MCL$_1$, and MCL$_6$).

lead ECG. This lead can be helpful in differentiating supraventricular tachycardia (SVT) from ventricular tachycardia (VT). To monitor using MCL_1, the brown lead should be in the V_1 position (the fourth intercostal space, to the right of the sternum). MCL_6 simulates V_6 of the twelve-lead ECG. To monitor in MCL_6, the brown lead should be in the V_6 position (the fifth intercostal space, at the midaxillary line).

Three-lead telemetry systems consist of a positive lead and a negative lead, with an additional neutral, or ground, lead. Lead I has a negative lead on the right arm and a positive lead on the left arm (Figure 6.10). Lead II has a negative lead on the right arm and a positive pole at the left lower abdomen (Figure 6.11). MCL_1 has a negative lead on the left arm, with the positive lead at the fourth intercostal space to the right of the sternum (Figure 6.12).

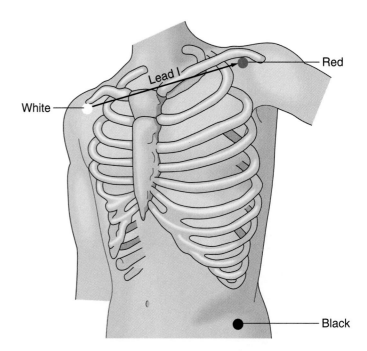

Figure 6.10 Three-lead telemetry (Lead I).

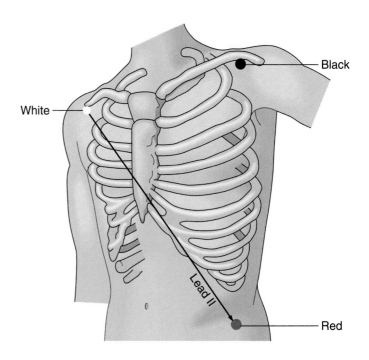

Figure 6.11 Three-lead telemetry (Lead II).

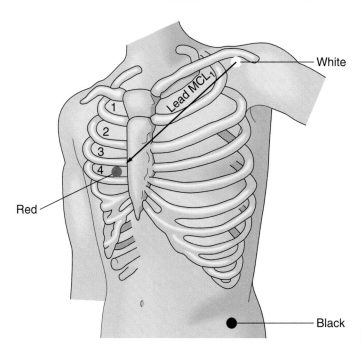

Figure 6.12 Three-lead telemetry (MCL$_1$).

The ECG Graph Paper

The paper that records ECG electrical activity is a grid. It records the time in seconds along the horizontal lines, and the voltage (the size of the activity) in millimeters (mm) along the vertical lines. The smallest size box represents 0.04 seconds. There are 1,500 small boxes in a minute (Figure 6.13).

Determining Heart Rate and Regularity

Heart rate can be calculated by different methods. The six-second interval method is the easiest way to calculate heart rate. It can be used if the heart rate is regular or irregular. There are usually short marks in 3-second intervals at the top of the ECG graph paper (Figure 6.14). The heart rate is calculated by counting the number of R waves in a 6-second interval and multiplying this number by 10. For example, in Figure 6.14, there are six QRS complexes in the 6-second interval.

$$6 \times 10 = 60 \text{ beats per minute}$$

The R-to-R interval method (Figure 6.15) can be used with regular rhythms and is very accurate. With this method, use calipers to measure the number of boxes between two consecutive R waves. For example, in Figure 6.15, there are fifteen small boxes between the R waves. Remember, there are 1,500 boxes in a minute.

$$\text{Heart rate} = \frac{1,500}{\text{No. of small boxes from R to R}}$$

$$\frac{1,500}{15} = 100 \text{ beats per minute}$$

Atrial rate can be determined by measuring the distance between consecutive waves using the same method.

Calipers can also be used to determine the regularity of the rhythm. The tips of the calipers are placed on the peaks of the R waves. Without moving the distance between the peaks of the calipers, the R-to-R intervals are compared across the ECG paper.

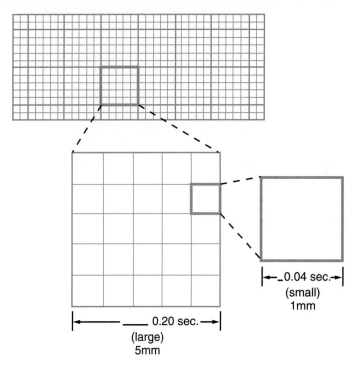

Figure 6.13 ECG graph paper measures electrical activity of the heart and the time it takes to complete each part of that activity.

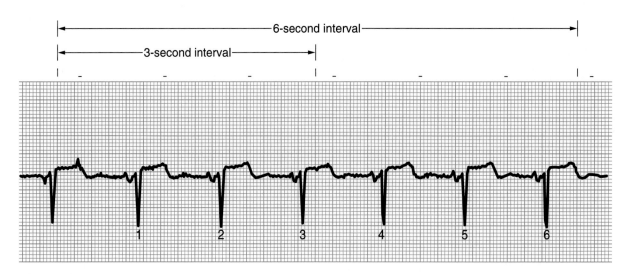

Figure 6.14 Three- and 6-second intervals.

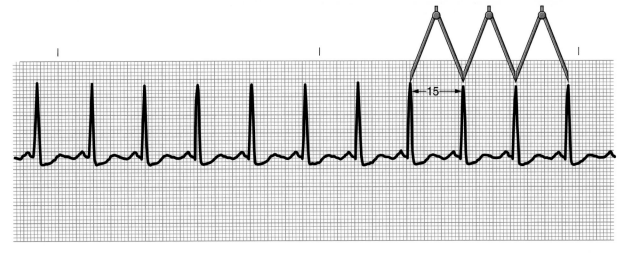

Figure 6.15 Heart rate = 1,500 ÷ (No. of small squares from R to R).

Pediatric and infant electrodes are available for children. Older adults, infants, and those patients with very sensitive skin might benefit from hyperallergenic electrodes. Check the skin of these patients for a rash or signs of irritation. Adult female patients who have very large breasts may need to have their left breast lifted to place the V_4 or V_5 electrode in the correct position.

Age-Specific Considerations

Key Concept

*T*he following might help you remember where the color leads are placed:
White = white is right (right chest below clavicle)
Black = opposite of right (left chest below clavicle)
Green = go! (accelerator pedal for driving a car—right upper iliac crest)
Red = stop! (brake on a car—left upper iliac crest)
Brown = fourth intercostal space to the right of the sternum

Steps for Setting Up Five-Lead Hardwire Monitoring

1. Wash hands.
2. Identify the correct patient.
3. Explain the procedure to the patient.
4. Assemble the equipment.
5. Prepare the patient's skin:
   a. Wash with soap and water; rinse and allow to dry. (Repeat with electrode change every 24 hours.)
   b. Clip excess hair if necessary.
6. Apply electrodes (use electrodes of the same brand and age):
   a. Check that the electrodes have fresh, moist gel.
   b. Attach the lead clip to the electrode.
   c. Apply the five electrodes, placing the lower electrodes just above the iliac crest bilaterally. Use the lead selector for the preferred lead.
7. Check for the characteristics of a good ECG signal:
   a. Stable baseline.
   b. QRS tall, narrow, and monophasic.
   c. T wave less than one-third the height of the R wave.
   d. P wave smaller than the T wave.
8. Obtain a rhythm strip:
   a. Observe for a good ECG signal.
   b. Locate and activate the record button on the monitor.
9. Document and report the results to the RN or preceptor.

Steps for Setting Up Three- or Five-Lead Telemetry Monitoring

1. Wash hands.
2. Identify the correct patient.
3. Explain the procedure to the patient.
4. Assemble the equipment.
5. Prepare the patient's skin:
   a. Wash with soap and water; rinse and allow to dry. (Repeat with electrode change every 24 hours.)
   b. Clip excess hair if necessary.
6. Apply electrodes (use electrodes of the same brand and age):
   a. Check that the electrodes have fresh, moist gel.
   b. Attach the lead clip to the electrode.
   c. Apply the five electrodes for Lead II and MCL_1, placing the lower electrodes just above the iliac crest bilaterally.
7. Operate the transmitter safely:
   a. Check the battery (zinc lasts 6 days versus 3 days for alkaline).
   b. Use a regular 9-volt alkaline battery when the patient showers.
   c. Demonstrate the disconnect/connect function.
   d. Instruct patient about how to use the nurse call button. (The button can run a strip from the room. The caregiver may teach the patient to use it in specific cases only; please use discretion!)
   e. Secure the transmitter safely in the patient's carrying pouch or holder.
8. Check for the characteristics of a good ECG signal:
   a. Stable baseline.
   b. QRS tall, narrow, and monophasic.
   c. T wave less than one-third the height of the R wave.
   d. P wave smaller than the T wave.
9. Obtain a rhythm strip:
   a. Observe for a good ECG signal.
   b. Locate and activate the record button on the monitor.
10. Document and report the results to the RN or preceptor.

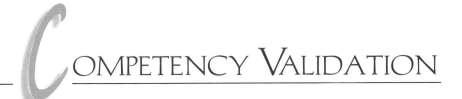

COMPETENCY VALIDATION

Skill: Setting Up Five-Lead Hardwire Monitoring

Name _____

Preceptor _____

Date _____

Competency Statement   Sets up five-lead hardwire monitoring while demonstrating correct technique.

Not Competent: _____ 1. Is <u>unable to state reason</u> for task and <u>needs instructions</u> to perform task.

_____ 2. Understands reason for task but <u>needs instructions</u> to perform task.

Competent: _____ 3. Understands reason for task and is able to perform task but <u>needs to increase speed.</u>

_____ 4. Understands reason for task and is able to perform task <u>proficiently.</u>

Performance Criteria

The caregiver demonstrates the ability to do the following:

_____ 1. Wash hands.

_____ 2. Identify the correct patient.

_____ 3. Explain the procedure to the patient.

_____ 4. Assemble the equipment.

_____ 5. Prepare the patient's skin:

_____ a. Wash with soap and water; rinse and allow to dry. (Repeat with electrode change every 24 hours.)

_____ b. Clip excess hair if necessary.

_____ 6. Apply electrodes (use electrodes of the same brand and age):

_____ a. Check that the electrodes have fresh, moist gel.

_____ b. Attach the lead clip to the electrode.

_____ c. Apply the five electrodes, placing the lower electrodes just above the iliac crest bilaterally. Use the lead selector for the preferred lead.

_____ 7. Check for the characteristics of a good ECG signal:

_____ a. Stable baseline.

_____ b. QRS tall, narrow, and monophasic.

_____ c. T wave less than one-third the height of the R wave.

_____ d. P wave smaller than the T wave.

_____ 8. Obtain a rhythm strip:

_____ a. Observe for a good ECG signal.

_____ b. Locate and activate the record button on the monitor.

_____ 9. Document and report the results to the RN or preceptor.

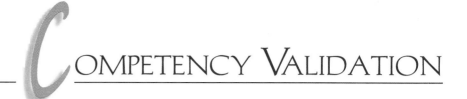

COMPETENCY VALIDATION

Setting Up Three- or Five-Lead Telemetry Monitoring

Name _____

Preceptor _____

Date _____

Competency Statement Sets up three- or five-lead telemetry monitoring while demonstrating correct technique.

Not Competent: _____ 1. Is <u>unable to state reason</u> for task and <u>needs instructions</u> to perform task.

_____ 2. Understands reason for task but <u>needs instructions</u> to perform task.

Competent: _____ 3. Understands reason for task and is able to perform but <u>needs to increase speed.</u>

_____ 4. Understands reason for task and is able to perform task <u>proficiently.</u>

Performance Criteria

The caregiver demonstrates the ability to do the following:

_____ 1. Wash hands.

_____ 2. Identify the correct patient.

_____ 3. Explain the procedure to the patient.

_____ 4. Assemble the equipment.

_____ 5. Prepare the patient's skin:

    _____ a. Wash with soap and water; rinse and allow to dry. (Repeat with electrode change every 24 hours.)

    _____ b. Clip excess hair if necessary.

_____ 6. Apply electrodes (use electrodes of the same brand and age):

    _____ a. Check that the electrodes have fresh, moist gel.

    _____ b. Attach the lead clip to the electrode.

    _____ c. Apply the five electrodes for Lead II and MCL_1, placing the lower electrodes just above the iliac crest bilaterally.

_____ 7. Operate the transmitter safely:

    _____ a. Check the battery (zinc lasts 6 days versus 3 days).

    _____ b. Use a regular 9-volt battery when the patient showers.

    _____ c. Check the disconnect/connect function.

    _____ d. Instruct patient about how to use the nurse call button. (The button runs a strip from the room. The caregiver may teach the patient to use it in specific cases only; please use discretion!)

    _____ e. Secure the transmitter safely in the patient's carrying pouch or holder.

_____ 8. Check for the characteristics of a good ECG signal:

    _____ a. Stable baseline.

    _____ b. QRS tall, narrow, and monophasic.

    _____ c. T wave less than one-third the height of the R wave.

    _____ d. P wave smaller than the T wave.

_____ 9. Obtain a rhythm strip:

    _____ a. Observe for a good ECG signal.

    _____ b. Locate and activate the record button on the monitor.

_____ 10. Document and report the results to the RN or preceptor.

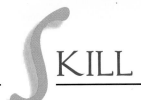

SKILL

Recognizing ECG Rhythms That Require RN Notification or Intervention

Purpose Early recognition and reporting of life-threatening arrhythmias are necessary for timely treatment by the health care team. It is important to identify a characteristic normal heart rhythm in order to differentiate it from abnormal rhythms (Table 6.1).

The caregiver demonstrates the ability to do the following:

Objectives

1. Recognize the components of normal sinus rhythm.

2. Recognize various arrhythmias.

3. Identify life-threatening arrhythmias.

Pertinent Points

- In *normal sinus rhythm,* the impulse is generated from the sinus node, which acts as the pacemaker of the heart. The heart rate is between 60 and 100 beats per minute, and the rhythm is regular. All intervals and waveforms are normal (Figure 6.16).

Rate:	60–100 beats per minute
Rhythm:	Regular
P wave:	Round, upright
PR interval:	0.12–0.20 seconds
QRS interval:	0.06–0.11 seconds

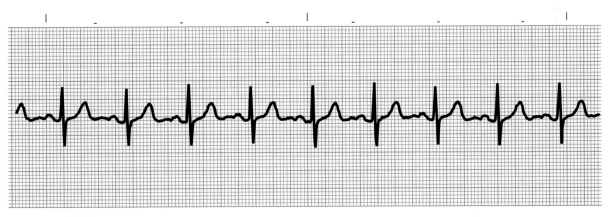

Figure 6.16 Normal sinus rhythm.

TABLE 6.1 ECG RHYTHM COMPARISON CHART

Rhythm	Atrial Rate (Beats Per Min.)	Atrial Rhythm	Ventricular Rate (Beats Per Min.)	Ventricular Rhythm	P Waves	PR Interval (Secs.)	QRS Interval (Secs.)
Normal sinus rhythm (SR)	60–100	Regular	60–100	Regular	Present; round, upright	0.12–0.20	0.06–0.11
Sinus bradycardia (SB)	Less than 60	Regular	Less than 60	Regular	Normal	Normal	Normal
Sinus tachycardia (ST)	Greater than 100	Regular	Greater than 100	Regular	Normal	Normal	Normal
Sinus arrhythmia	60–100	Irregular	60–100	Irregular	Normal	Normal	Normal
Sinus arrest	Normal to slow	Irregular with pauses	Normal to slow	Irregular with pauses	Absent during pause	Normal with conducted beat; absent with pause	Normal
Wandering atrial pacemaker	Normal to slow	Irregular	Normal to slow	Irregular	Vary in size and shape; might be absent	Varies	Normal
Premature atrial contraction (PAC)	Depends on underlying rhythm	Irregular due to PAC	Depends on underlying rhythm	Irregular due to PAC	Differs from that of sinus beat	Normal but differs from sinus interval	Normal
Atrial fibrillation	Varies; F waves very rapid, up to 360 per minute	Irregularly irregular	Varies	Irregular	Absent; F (fibrillation) waves	None	Usually normal
Atrial flutter	250–400	Regular	60–150	Usually regular	Absent; F (flutter) waves	None	Normal
Premature junctional contraction (PJC)	Depends on underlying rhythm	Irregular due to premature beat	Depends on underlying rhythm	Irregular due to premature beat	Might be absent, inverted, before or after QRS	Less than 0.12	Normal
Junctional rhythm	If seen, atrial rate is equal to ventricular rate	Regular, if seen	40–60	Regular	Might be absent, inverted, before or after QRS	Less than 0.12	Normal
Paroxysmal supraventricular tachycardia (PSVT)	150–250	Regular; might not be able to determine atrial activity	150–250	Regular	Might be concealed in previous T wave	Might be impossible to measure	Normal
First-degree AV block	Depends on underlying rhythm	Depends on underlying rhythm	Depends on underlying rhythm	Depends on underlying rhythm	Normal	Greater than 0.20	Normal
Second-degree block—Mobitz I (Wenckebach)	Usually normal	Regular	Slower than atrial	Irregular	Normal shape	Progressive lengthening until QRS is dropped	Normal

Rhythm	Atrial Rate (Beats Per Min.)	Atrial Rhythm	Ventricular Rate (Beats Per Min.)	Ventricular Rhythm	P Waves	PR Interval (Secs.)	QRS Interval (Secs.)
Second-degree block—Mobitz II	Normal	Regular	Slower than atrial	Irregular	Normal	Consistent for conducted beats	Greater than 0.12
Third-degree block	Usually normal	Regular; no relationship to ventricular rhythm	Slower than atrial	Regular; no relationship to atrial rhythm	Normal	No relationship to QRS	Greater than 0.12
Premature ventricular contraction (PVC)	Depends on underlying rhythm	Irregular due to premature beat	Depends on underlying rhythm	Irregular due to premature beat	Absent	Absent	Greater than 0.12; wide and bizarre
Ventricular tachycardia (V Tach)	None	None	150–250	Regular	Absent	Absent	Greater than 0.12
Ventricular fibrillation (V Fib)	Cannot be determined	None	Cannot be determined	Chaotic	Absent	Absent	Cannot be determined
Asystole	None	None	None	None	Absent	Absent	Absent
Idioventricular rhythm	None	None	20–45	Might be irregular	Absent	Absent	Greater than 0.12; wide and bizarre
Ventricular paced rhythm	None	None	Set on the pacemaker	Preset backup rate—Regular	Usually absent	Not measured	Greater than 0.12

- In *sinus bradycardia,* the impulse originates from the SA node, as in normal sinus rhythm, but the rate is slower. The decrease in heart rate is significant when the patient relates symptoms associated with this decrease, such as a decrease in systolic blood pressure, dizziness, light-headedness, or syncope (fainting). Sinus bradycardia is normal during sleep and in trained athletes (Figure 6.17).

Rate:	Less than 60 beats per minute
Rhythm:	Regular
P wave:	Normal
PR interval:	Normal
QRS interval:	Normal

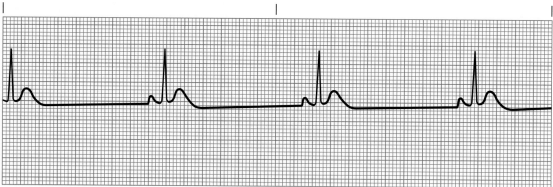

Figure 6.17 Sinus bradycardia.

- The onset and termination of *sinus tachycardia,* or rapid heart rate, are usually gradual. The impulse originates from the SA node. Sinus tachycardia can be a normal response to exercise or emotion. In healthy individuals, it is an arrhythmia that usually does not need to be treated (Figure 6.18).

Rate:	Greater than 100 beats per minute
Rhythm:	Regular
P wave:	Normal
PR interval:	Normal
QRS interval:	Normal

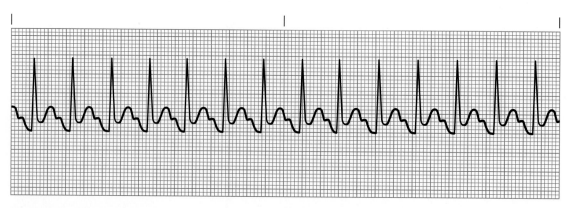

Figure 6.18 Sinus tachycardia.

- *Sinus arrhythmia,* or irregular rhythm, is commonly related to respiration. It is normally seen in children, young adults, and the elderly. The heart rate increases with inspiration and decreases with expiration (Figure 6.19).

Rate:	Usually 60–100 beats per minute
Rhythm:	Irregular
P wave:	Normal
PR interval:	Normal
QRS interval:	Normal

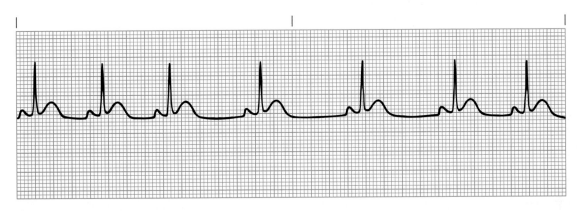

Figure 6.19 Sinus arrhythmia.

- *Sinus arrest* occurs when the electrical impulse is not generated by the SA node, and a P wave is not seen. A pause in the rhythm will be seen until the SA node fires another beat or an escape rhythm is generated by another area of the heart in response to this pause. The length of the pause is not an interval of the normal R-to-R rhythm (Figure 6.20).

Rate:	Usually 60–100 beats per minute, but might be slower if pauses are frequent
Rhythm:	Irregular when the pauses occur
P wave:	Normal with the conducted beats; absent with the pauses
PR interval:	Normal with the conducted beats; absent with the pauses
QRS interval:	Normal

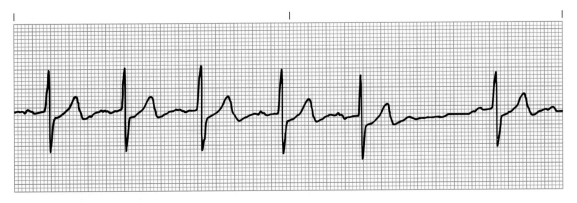

Figure 6.20 Sinus arrest.

- *Wandering atrial pacemaker* occurs when the pacemaker of the heart moves from the SA node to the atria and to the AV node. The rate slows as the impulse shifts from a higher area of the heart, such as the SA node, to a slower area of the heart, such as the AV node. This arrhythmia does not usually require treatment (Figure 6.21).

Rate:	Usually 60–100 beats per minute, but might be slower
Rhythm:	Irregular as impulse shifts
P wave:	Shape changes as pacemaker changes from one site to another; might even be absent when the beat originates within AV node
PR interval:	Varies
QRS interval:	Normal

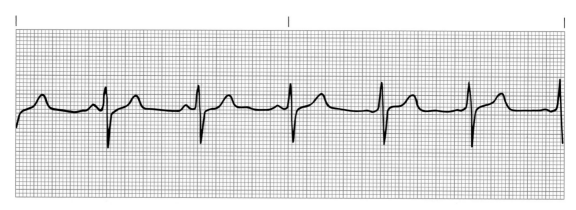

Figure 6.21 Wandering atrial pacemaker.

- *A premature atrial contraction (PAC)* occurs when an impulse originates from outside the SA node and occurs somewhere in the atria. The impulse occurs earlier than the next expected sinus beat and is therefore considered to be premature. Single PACS can occur in healthy hearts and do not require treatment. In patients with heart disease, multiple PACS can precipitate other dysrhythmias, such as atrial fibrillation, atrial flutter, and paroxysmal (sudden onset) atrial tachycardia (PAT). Three or more PACS in a row are considered to be PAT. Heart rates with PAT can be between 150 and 250 (Figure 6.22).

Rate:	Depends on underlying rhythm
Rhythm:	Irregular with the PACS
P wave:	With the PAC can be a different shape from the sinus P wave
PR interval:	Within normal limits but usually different from the sinus PR interval
QRS interval:	Normal

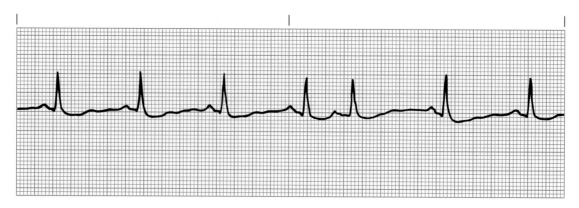

Figure 6.22 Premature atrial contractions.

- *Atrial fibrillation* has a characteristic of being "irregularly irregular." The pacemaker of the heart comes from multiple sites in the atria. This activity is erratic, causing the baseline to appear very irregular and chaotic. The F waves, or atrial activity, usually do not resemble normal P waves. The AV node randomly conducts some of these impulses down through the rest of the conduction pathway, causing the irregular rhythm (Figure 6.23).

Rate:	Ventricular rate can vary from bradycardia to tachycardia; F waves occur very rapidly, up to 360 per minute
Rhythm:	Irregularly irregular
P wave:	Absent; F waves seen (chaotic baseline)
PR interval:	None
QRS interval:	Usually normal, but can be wide if a conduction disturbance is present

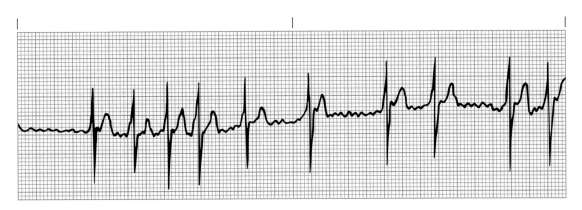

Figure 6.23 Atrial fibrillation.

- *Atrial flutter* is a repetitive firing of a stimulus in the atria. The rhythm of the firing is regular and creates an unmistakable "sawtooth" monitor pattern. The origin of this focus is not from the sinus node, but from another area in the atria. The ventricles are unable to respond to each atrial stimulus. The AV node filters some of the atrial stimuli and sends only some of the stimuli on to the ventricles to be conducted. Typically, the conduction is expressed as a ratio of the number of atrial beats compared to ventricular conducted beats— for example, 2:1 (two P waves preceding every QRS), 3:1 (three P waves to every QRS), and so on (Figure 6.24).

Rate:	Ventricular rate is usually 60–150 beats per minute; flutter waves occur very rapidly, up to 400 per minute
Rhythm:	Usually regular
P wave:	Absent; flutter waves seen ("sawtooth" baseline)
PR interval:	None
QRS interval:	Normal

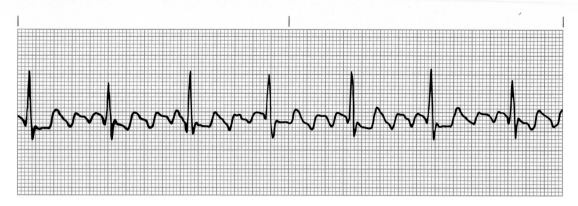

Figure 6.24 Atrial flutter.

- *A premature junctional contraction* is a beat that originates at the AV junction (AV node). The beat comes before the next expected regular beat. Because the stimulus is not initiated at the sinus node, it does not have a characteristic P wave. Instead, there might be no P wave at all, or the P wave may look inverted or biphasic (like an S on its side). The P wave might be seen in the ST segment (Figure 6.25).

Rate:	Depends on underlying rhythm
Rhythm:	Irregular due to premature beat
P wave:	Might be absent, inverted, before or after QRS
PR interval:	Less than 0.12 seconds
QRS interval:	Normal

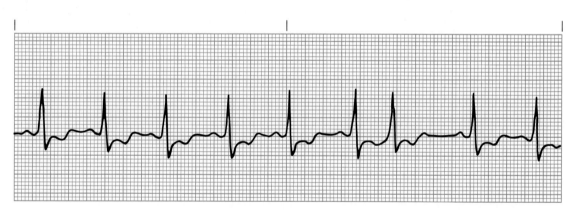

Figure 6.25 Premature junctional contractions.

- *A junctional rhythm* is a characteristically slow rhythm that originates at the AV junction. In this rhythm, the AV junction assumes the role of pacemaker for the heart. P waves are absent, inverted, or biphasic. The QRS is usually narrow. The rate of a junctional rhythm is usually 40 to 60 beats per minute. A junctional rate is considered accelerated if the rate falls between 60 and 100 beats per minute (Figure 6.26).

Rate:	Ventricular rate is usually 40–60 beats per minute
Rhythm:	Regular
P wave:	Might be absent, inverted, before or after the QRS
PR interval:	Less than 0.12 seconds
QRS interval:	Normal

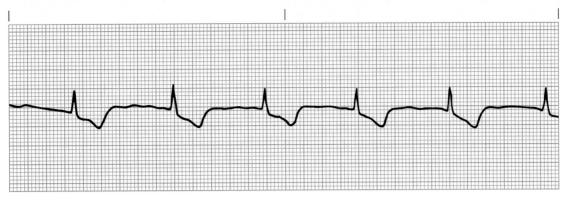

Figure 6.26 Junctional rhythm.

- *Paroxysmal supraventricular tachycardia* describes a narrow QRS complex rhythm that originates above the ventricles but not from the SA node. The rate exceeds 100 beats per minute, and the rhythm is usually regular (Figure 6.27).

Rate:	Ventricular rate is 150–250; might be unable to determine atrial rate
Rhythm:	Ventricular rhythm is regular
P wave:	Might be concealed in previous T wave
PR interval:	Might be impossible to measure
QRS interval:	Normal

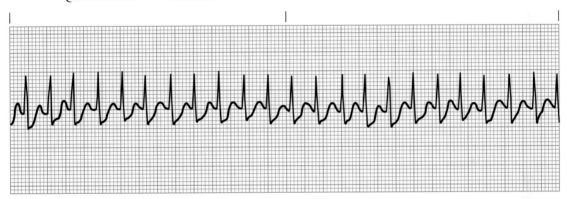

Figure 6.27 Paroxysmal supraventricular tachycardia.

- *A first-degree AV block* exists when the length of the PR interval exceeds 0.20 seconds (five small ECG boxes) (Figure 6.28).

Rate:	Depends on underlying rhythm
Rhythm:	Depends on underlying rhythm
P wave:	Normal
PR interval:	Greater than 0.20 seconds
QRS interval:	Normal

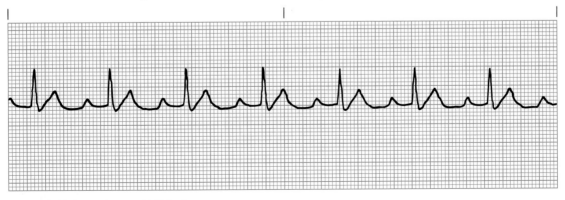

Figure 6.28 First-degree AV block.

- *Second-degree block—Mobitz I (Wenckebach)* is described as a rhythm in which the PR interval progressively lengthens until a P wave does not generate a QRS. The cycle then resumes with progressively lengthening PR intervals until another P wave does not generate a QRS (Figure 6.29).

Rate:	Ventricular is slower than atrial; atrial is usually normal
Rhythm:	Ventricular is irregular; atrial is regular
P wave:	Normal
PR interval:	Progressive lengthening until QRS is dropped
QRS interval:	Normal

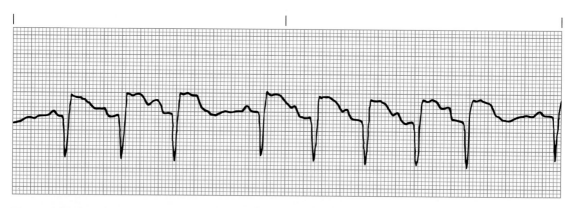

Figure 6.29 Second-degree AV block—Mobitz I (Wenckebach).

- *Second-degree block—Mobitz II* is characterized by a prolonged PR interval with a periodically dropped QRS (P wave but no QRS). The PR interval does not progressively increase, as seen in Mobitz I (Wenckebach). The R-to-R interval with the conducted beat is consistently the same. The QRS is usually wide due to a conduction disturbance in the bundle of His (Figure 6.30).

Rate:	Ventricular is slower than atrial; atrial is normal
Rhythm:	Ventricular is irregular; atrial is regular
P wave:	Normal
PR interval:	Consistent for conducted beats
QRS interval:	Greater than 0.12 seconds

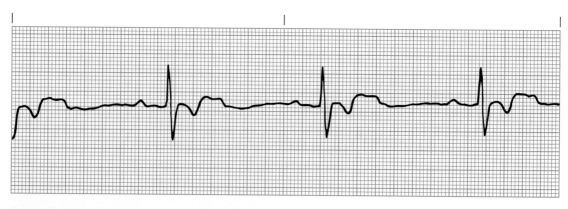

Figure 6.30 Second-degree AV block—Mobitz II.

- In *third-degree block,* the atria and ventricles beat in a regular rhythm but are totally independent of one another. The ventricles beat at a rate slower than the atria. The rhythm can be life-threatening if the ventricular rate is not sufficient to maintain cardiac output (Figure 6.31).

Rate: Ventricular is slower than atrial; atrial is usually normal
Rhythm: Both ventricular and atrial are regular but totally independent
P wave: Normal
PR interval: No relationship of P wave to QRS
QRS interval: Greater than 0.12 seconds

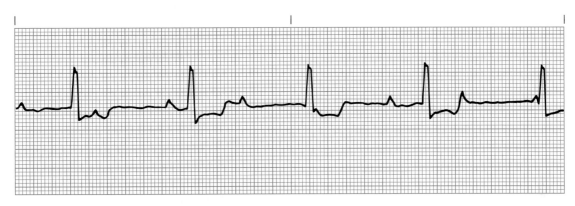

Figure 6.31 Third-degree block.

- *Premature ventricular contractions (PVCs)* originate from stimuli in an irritable wall of the ventricle. The QRS complex is wide and not preceded by a P wave. The stimulus comes before the next expected regular beat and is usually followed by a compensatory pause. This compensatory pause is defined as the time the sinus node waits after the premature beat before initiating the next sinus beat on its previous schedule (Figure 6.32).

Rate: Depends on underlying rhythm
Rhythm: Irregular due to premature beat
P wave: Absent
PR interval: Absent
QRS interval: Greater than 0.12 seconds; wide and bizarre

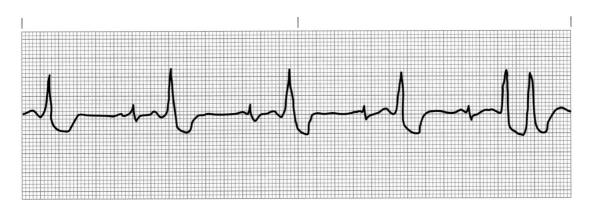

Figure 6.32 Premature ventricular contractions.

- *Ventricular tachycardia* is a rapid series of beats (usually greater than 150 beats per minute) initiated in the ventricle. This rapid firing might not leave sufficient time for the ventricles to fill with blood after each beat, and therefore some beats might not be palpated as peripheral pulses. Left untreated, ventricular tachycardia can quickly lead to ventricular fibrillation, a life-threatening arrhythmia (Figure 6.33).

Rate:	Ventricular is 150–250 beats per minute; no atrial beats seen
Rhythm:	Regular
P wave:	Absent
PR interval:	Absent
QRS interval:	Greater than 0.12 seconds

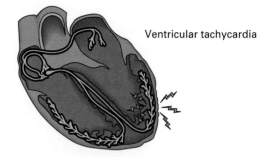

Ventricular tachycardia

ECG tracing of ventricular tachycardia

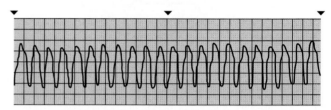

Figure 6.33 Ventricular tachycardia.

- *Ventricular fibrillation* is a life-threatening arrhythmia characterized by a quivering of the ventricles. This is displayed as chaotic fibrillatory waves on the ECG monitor. No effective ventricular contractions take place; no peripheral pulses are felt; and if left untreated, the patient dies (Figure 6.34).

Rate:	Cannot be determined
Rhythm:	None
P wave:	Absent
PR interval:	Absent
QRS interval:	Cannot be determined

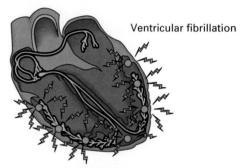

Ventricular fibrillation

Chaotic electrical discharge as seen on an ECG tracing

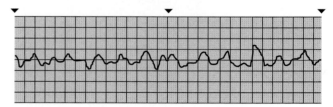

Figure 6.34 Ventricular fibrillation.

- *Asystole* is defined as an absence of atrial or ventricular contractions. There is a characteristic flat line pattern on the monitor. Before assuming asystole, the caregiver must always assess for loose leads or other mechanical problems that might imitate asystole. True asystole is a life-threatening arrhythmia and must be treated immediately. *Ventricular asystole* is characterized by an absence of ventricular complexes, although P waves might be present (Figure 6.35).

Rate:	None
Rhythm:	None
P wave:	Absent
PR interval:	Absent
QRS interval:	Absent

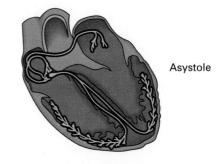

Asystole

ECG tracing of asystole

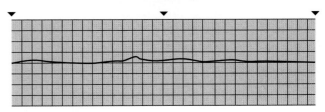

Figure 6.35 Asystole.

- An *idioventricular rhythm* is defined as a rhythm in which the ventricles assume the role of pacemaker for the heart. The complexes are wide and slow, and no P waves are seen. The normal idioventricular rate is 20 to 45 beats per minute. This rhythm is often associated with the dying heart (Figure 6.36).

Rate:	Ventricular rate is 20–45 beats per minute; no atrial rate
Rhythm:	Might be irregular
P wave:	Absent
PR interval:	Absent
QRS interval:	Greater than 0.12 seconds; wide and bizarre

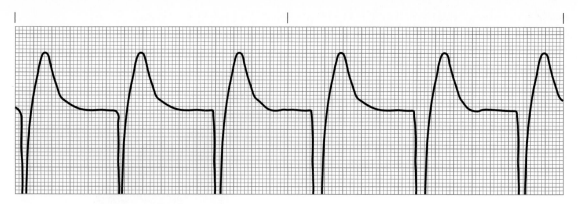

Figure 6.36 Idioventricular rhythm.

- *Ventricular paced rhythm* is initiated by an artificial pacemaker source. A wire is implanted in the right ventricle and attached to a pacemaker generator. The pacemaker beats at a set backup rate unless it senses that the heart has its own natural beats. Characteristic spikes are noted on the ECG monitor; these are followed by QRS complexes (Figure 6.37).

Rate:	When paced, the ventricular rate is the rate set on the pacemaker generator
Rhythm:	Paced beats are regular
P wave:	Usually absent in paced beats
PR interval:	Not measured

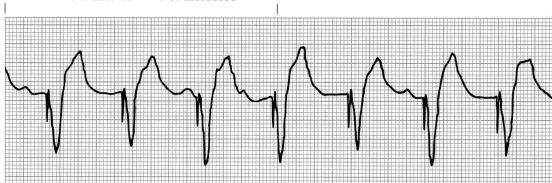

Figure 6.37 Ventricular paced rhythm.

Age-Specific Considerations

Heart rates might vary for children of different ages and still be considered within the normal ranges (Table 6.2). In infants, *sinus tachycardia* is usually associated with heart rates of less than 200 beats per minute. *Supraventricular tachycardia (SVT)* in infants is generally greater than 230 beats per minute. *Ventricular tachycardia* is uncommon in children unless there is structural disease, electrolyte abnormalities, or acidosis present. *Sinus bradycardia and AV blocks* are the most common terminal rhythms in children.

TABLE 6.2 NORMAL PEDIATRIC HEART RATES

AGE	AWAKE HEART RATE	AVERAGE HEART RATE	SLEEPING HEART RATE
Newborn–3 months	85–205	140	80–160
3 months–2 years	100–190	130	75–160
2 years–10 years	60–140	80	60–90
> 10 years	60–100	75	50–90

The ECG machine not only records the electrical activity of the heart, but it can also record extra electrical activity or muscle movement. Loose electrodes can cause erratic electrical interference on the ECG monitor (Figure 6.38). Ensure that all leads are securely attached, and change electrode patches if necessary to ensure good contact. Sixty-cycle interference appears on the monitor as a tall band throughout all or some parts of the cardiac complex (Figure 6.39). It is caused by electrical interference in the area. Resolve this artifact by disconnecting electrical devices one at a time from the outlet until sixty-cycle interference is gone. The ground wire of that electrical device needs repair.

1. Complete the ECG competency test.
2. Review your answers with the preceptor.

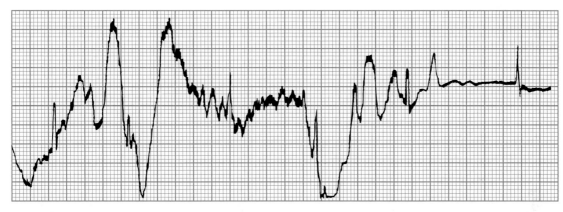

Figure 6.38 Artifact.

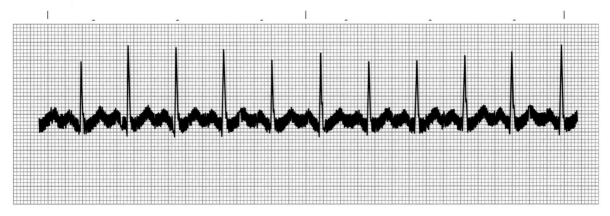

Figure 6.39 Sixty-cycle interference.

ECG Competency

Name _____

Preceptor _____

Date _____

Directions: Identify the ventricular rate, PR interval, and QRS interval for each of the following tracings. (Each question is worth 2 points.)

1.
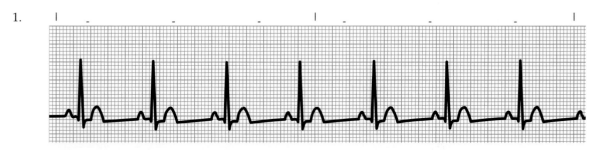

Figure 6.A

Ventricular rate: _____   PR interval: _____   QRS interval: _____

2.
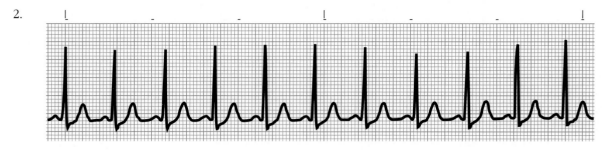

Figure 6.B

Ventricular rate: _____   PR interval: _____   QRS interval: _____

Directions: Write your interpretation of each of the following tracings on the corresponding line. Be sure to write complete interpretations. (Each question is worth 1 point.)

3.
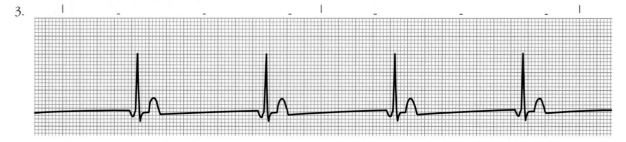

Figure 6.C

Interpretation: _____

4.

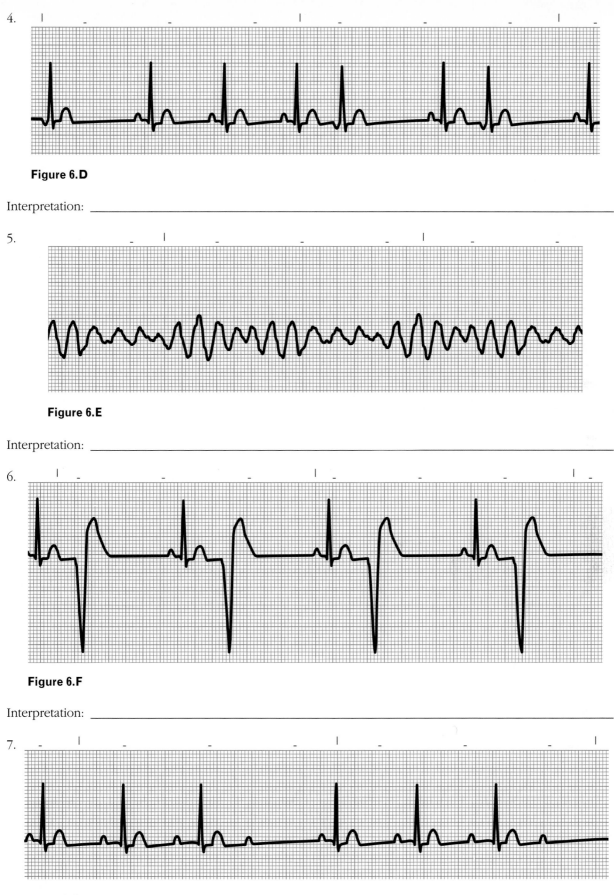

Figure 6.D

Interpretation: _____

5.

Figure 6.E

Interpretation: _____

6.

Figure 6.F

Interpretation: _____

7.

Figure 6.G

Interpretation: _____

8.

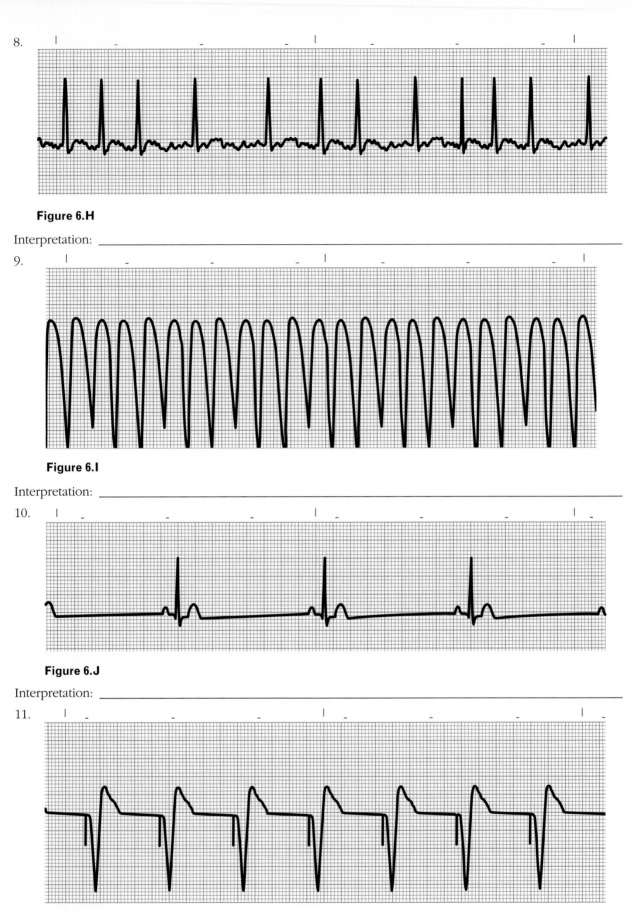

Figure 6.H

Interpretation: _____

9.

Figure 6.I

Interpretation: _____

10.

Figure 6.J

Interpretation: _____

11.

Figure 6.K

Interpretation: _____

12.

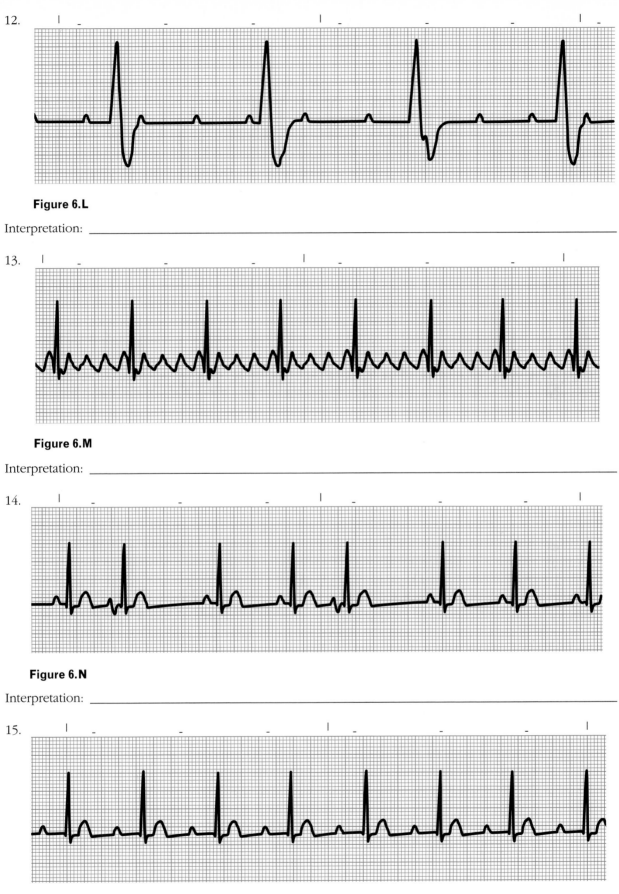

Figure 6.L

Interpretation: _____

13.

Figure 6.M

Interpretation: _____

14.

Figure 6.N

Interpretation: _____

15.

Figure 6.O

Interpretation: _____

16.

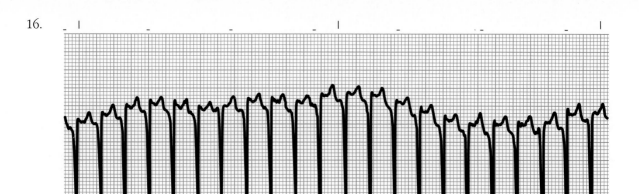

Figure 6.P

Interpretation: _____

17.

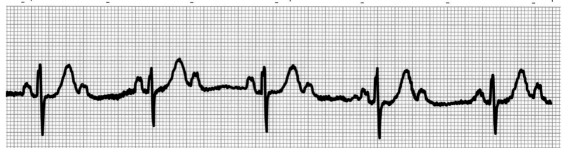

Figure 6.Q

Interpretation: _____

18.

Figure 6.R

Interpretation: _____

Test Answers

_____ 1. Rate: 70, PR: 0.16, QRS: 0.08
_____ 2. Rate: 110, PR: 0.12, QRS: 0.08
_____ 3. Junctional rhythm, rate: 40
_____ 4. Sinus rhythm with premature junctional contractions, rate: 70
_____ 5. Ventricular fibrillation
_____ 6. Sinus rhythm with bigeminal premature ventricular contractions, rate: 70
_____ 7. Second-degree AV Block—Mobitz I (Wenckebach), rate: 50
_____ 8. Atrial fibrillation, rate: 110
_____ 9. Ventricular tachycardia, rate: 220
_____ 10. Sinus bradycardia, rate: 30
_____ 11. 100 percent ventricular paced rhythm, rate: 70
_____ 12. Third-degree heart block (complete heart block), rate: 40
_____ 13. Atrial flutter (4:1), rate: 70
_____ 14. Sinus rhythm with premature atrial contractions, rate: 70
_____ 15. Sinus rhythm with first-degree AV block (PR .30), rate: 80
_____ 16. Supraventricular tachycardia, rate: 220 (narrow QRS)
_____ 17. Sinus tachycardia, rate: 140
_____ 18. Second-degree AV block—Mobitz II (2:1), rate: 50

SKILL

Performing Twelve-Lead ECG Monitoring

Purpose   The twelve-lead ECG machine is a portable bedside device used to record six bipolar (limb) leads and six chest (precordial) leads for a complete electrocardiogram (Figure 6.40). Waveforms are recorded on specialized ECG paper and are interpreted by a physician.

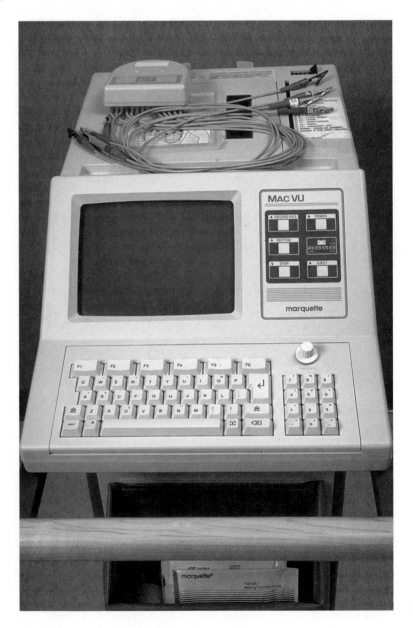

Figure 6.40 Portable twelve-lead ECG machine.

The caregiver demonstrates the ability to do the following:

1. Gather the correct supplies.

2. Communicate using a style that reduces the patient's anxiety.

3. Locate the correct sites and prepare the patient's skin for a twelve-lead ECG.

4. Identify the characteristics of a good ECG signal.

5. Obtain an ECG using a portable machine.

6. Report the results of the procedure to the RN or preceptor.

Augmented Made larger; increased.

Bigeminy The state of having an ectopic beat that occurs every other beat.

Caliper A tool used to assist in measuring heart rate and rhythm on an ECG strip.

Couplets Two abnormal beats that occur in a row.

Ectopic Situated somewhere other than the normal place.

Ectopy Abnormal beats.

Electrode Gel A gelatinous substance that is used with the ECG electrodes to transmit a good-quality signal to the ECG monitor.

Hardwire Monitoring A monitoring system by which the patient is physically connected to a monitoring device that displays the ECG rhythm at the bedside.

Isoelectric Line The flat area of an ECG where no electrical impulse is detected. Also called baseline.

Multifocal Pertaining to two or more ectopic beats that look different from one another.

Premature Beat A cardiac contraction that occurs before the next normal beat is expected.

Rhythm Strip A long (6- to 12-second) ECG recording of one or more leads during cardiac monitoring.

Stylus The needlelike instrument that writes the heart rhythm onto ECG paper.

Telemetry A system in which the patient is attached to ECG leads and a portable transmitter, which sends radio signals to a central monitor, where the patient's ECG can be viewed.

Unifocal Pertaining to two or more beats that look alike.

Twelve-lead ECG machine • Disposable adhesive-tab electrodes • Soap and water • Clippers to remove hair (if needed)

- The twelve-lead ECG machine is used to look at the heart from several different views simultaneously. Information gained during twelve-lead monitoring can be used to diagnose the cardiac rhythm, identify arrhythmias and conduction disturbances, and determine the presence and location of previous or recent myocardial infarctions.

- Patient information—such as name, age, height, weight, ethnic background, and current cardiac medications—is entered into the machine's computer. The physician who reads the ECG will use this information in formulating an interpretation.

- A disposable adhesive tab is placed on the clean, dry skin of each forearm and lower leg and at six points across the chest (Figures 6.41 and 6.42). The tabs are connected to the lead wires of the twelve-lead ECG machine.

- Instruct the patient to breathe normally and lie still while the ECG data are collected. Any movement will appear as artifact on the ECG paper.

- When all of the connections are intact, push the record button.

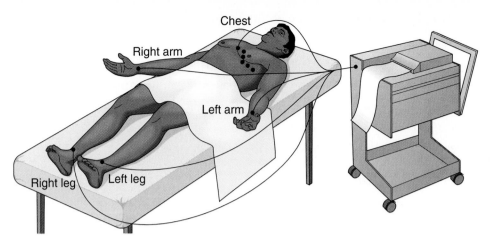

Chest

Right arm

Left arm

Right leg   Left leg

Figure 6.41 Twelve-lead ECG.

Lead V$_1$ The electrode is at the fourth intercostal space just to the right of the sternum.

Lead V$_2$ The electrode is at the fourth intercostal space just to the left of the sternum.

Lead V$_3$ The electrode is at the line midway between leads V$_2$ and V$_4$.

Lead V$_4$ The electrode is at the midclavicular line in the fifth interspace.

Lead V$_5$ The electrode is at the anterior axillary line at the same level as lead V$_4$.

Lead V$_6$ The electrode is at the midaxillary line at the same level as lead V$_4$.

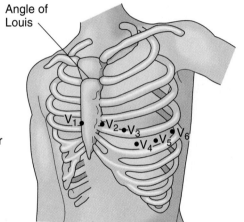

Angle of Louis

V_1 V_2 V_3 V_4 V_5 V_6

Figure 6.42 Proper placement of the precordial leads.

- The characteristics of a good signal include a relatively flat baseline and no artifact. If a poor signal exists, check that the patient is lying still and that all leads and tabs are securely placed.
- The machine will write the recorded electrical waveforms onto the specialized machine paper (Figures 6.43 to 6.49). The data might also be recorded onto an internal disk for transmittal to a central collection site where they will be read by a cardiologist.
- Once the recording process is complete, disconnect the lead wires, and remove and discard the tabs.

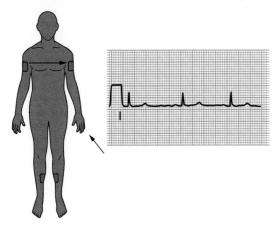

Figure 6.43 Lead I reads from the right arm to the left arm and looks similar to this.

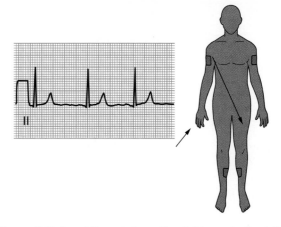

Figure 6.44 Lead II reads from the right arm to the left leg and looks similar to this.

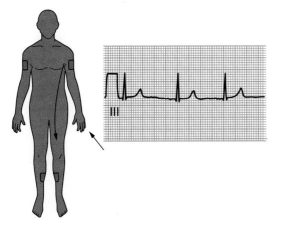

Figure 6.45 Lead III reads from the left arm to the left leg and looks similar to this.

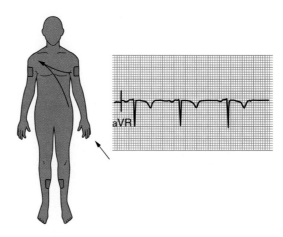

Figure 6.46 Lead aVR reads across the heart to the right arm and looks similar to this.

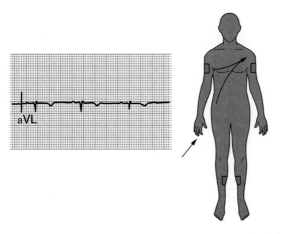

Figure 6.47 Lead aVL reads across the heart to the left arm and looks similar to this.

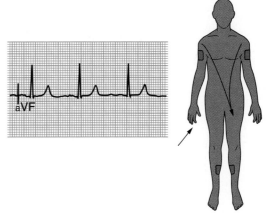

Figure 6.48 Lead aVF reads across the heart toward the feet and looks similar to this.

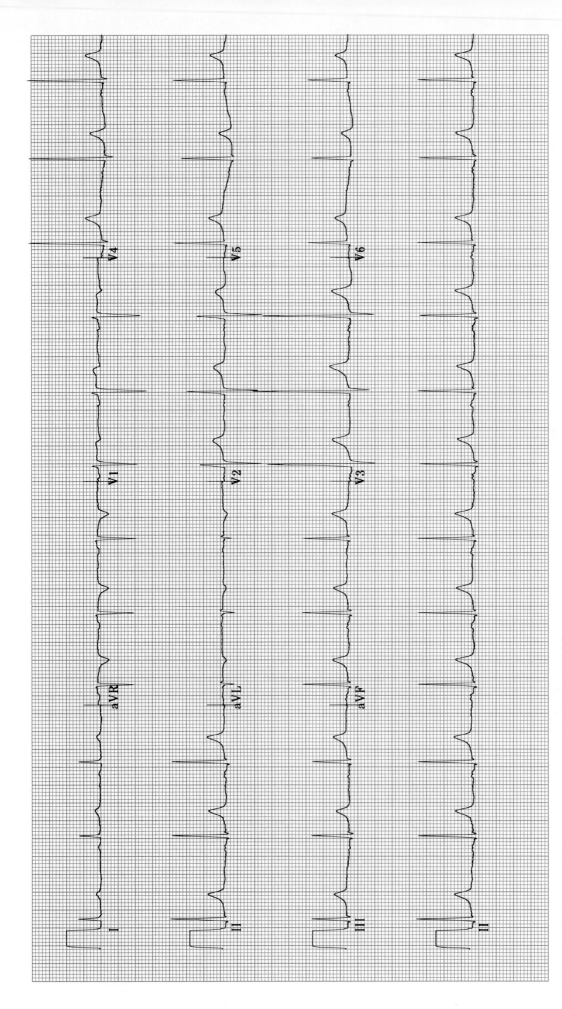

Figure 6.49 Tracing of a patient with a normal twelve-lead ECG.

You might need to cut the tabs in half (or use pediatric tabs) for small children and infants. Older adults, infants, and those patients with very sensitive skin might benefit from hyperallergenic electrodes. Check the skin of these patients for a rash or signs of irritation.

*B*e sure to record patient information accurately—including name, age, height, weight, ethnic background, and current cardiac medications—as you enter it into the machine's computer. The physician who reads the ECG will use this information in formulating an interpretation.

1. Wash hands.
2. Identify the correct patient.
3. Explain the procedure to the patient.
4. Assemble the equipment.
5. Prepare the patient's skin:
   a. Wash with soap and water; rinse and allow to dry. The tabs must be placed on clean, dry skin.
   b. Clip excess hair if necessary.
6. Apply electrode tabs and leads:
   a. Place a tab on each lower arm and lower leg. Do not put tabs over broken or irritated skin or directly over bony areas.
   b. Apply six chest tabs over the sternum and around the left side of the chest (Figure 6.42).
   c. Securely attach the corresponding lead clip to each electrode tab. All of the lead clips are color-coded and labeled.
7. Enter patient data into the ECG machine, using the keyboard.

8. Press the "Record ECG" button. Remind the patient to lie still until the machine has recorded the information.
9. Check for the characteristics of a good ECG signal:
   a. Stable baseline.
   b. QRS tall, narrow, and monophasic.
   c. T wave less than one-third the height of the R wave.
   d. P wave smaller than the T wave.
10. Obtain a rhythm strip:
    a. Observe for a good ECG signal.
    b. Locate and activate the "Rhythm Strip" button on the monitor.
11. Discontinue the setup:
    a. Disconnect the lead clips from the tabs, and return them to the cart.
    b. Carefully peel the leads from the chest and limbs, and discard.
12. Document and report the results to the RN or preceptor.

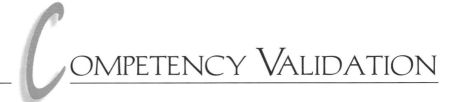

COMPETENCY VALIDATION

Skill: Performing Twelve-Lead ECG Monitoring

Name _____

Preceptor _____

Date _____

Competency Statement Performs twelve-lead ECG monitoring while demonstrating correct technique.

Not Competent: _____ 1. Is <u>unable to state reason</u> for task and <u>needs instructions</u> to perform task.

_____ 2. Understands reason for task but <u>needs instructions</u> to perform task.

Competent: _____ 3. Understands reason for task and is able to perform task but <u>needs to increase speed.</u>

_____ 4. Understands reason for task and is able to perform task <u>proficiently.</u>

Performance Criteria

The caregiver demonstrates the ability to do the following:

_____ 1. Wash hands.

_____ 2. Identify the correct patient.

_____ 3. Explain the procedure to the patient.

_____ 4. Assemble the equipment.

_____ 5. Prepare the patient's skin.

    _____ a. If necessary, wash with soap and water; rinse and allow to dry. The tabs must be placed on clean, dry skin.

    _____ b. Clip excess hair if necessary.

_____ 6. Apply electrode tabs and leads:

    _____ a. Place a tab on each lower arm and lower leg. Do not put tabs over broken or irritated skin or directly over bony areas.

    _____ b. Apply six chest tabs over the sternum and around the left side of the chest.

    _____ c. Securely attach the corresponding lead clip to each electrode tab. All of the lead clips are color-coded and labeled.

_____ 7. Enter patient data into the ECG machine, using the keyboard.

_____ 8. Press the "Record ECG" button. Remind the patient to lie still until the machine has recorded the information.

_____ 9. Check for the characteristics of a good ECG signal:

    _____ a. Stable baseline.

    _____ b. QRS tall, narrow, and monophasic.

    _____ c. T wave less than one-third the height of the R wave.

    _____ d. P wave smaller than the T wave.

_____ 10. Obtain a rhythm strip:

    _____ a. Observe for a good ECG signal.

    _____ b. Locate and activate the "Rhythm Strip" button on the monitor.

_____ 11. Discontinue the setup:

    _____ a. Disconnect the lead clips from the tabs, and return them to the cart.

    _____ b. Carefully peel the leads from the chest and limbs, and discard.

_____ 12. Document and report the results to the RN or preceptor.

THE PATIENT WITH AN ARTERIAL LINE

Arterial catheters are inserted for patients who need close blood pressure monitoring or frequent blood draws. Generally, a physician places an intravenous catheter into the radial artery and sutures the catheter in place. Although most arterial catheters are placed in the radial artery, an alternate site for placement of the catheter is in the femoral artery. Once placed, the catheter is covered with a sterile occlusive dressing and is immediately connected to a monitoring system (Figure 6.50). The system includes five parts: the transducer, the fluid-filled pressure tubing, the solution, a pressure bag, and the intraflow device.

Pertinent Points: Advantages and Risks of an Arterial Line

The use of an arterial line provides several advantages, including continuous accurate measurement of blood pressure, detection of blood pressure trends, and convenient access for blood draws. Disadvantages, however, do exist. The risk of bleeding, embolism, vessel and tissue damage, and infection must be considered.
To minimize the risk of bleeding,

- Consistently maintain the pressure at 300 mmHg in the pressure bag.
- Ensure that all connections and stopcocks are positioned properly and securely.
- Set alarm limits to warn of decreases in blood pressure.

To avoid embolism and vessel or tissue damage,

- Notify the RN of any patient complaints of pain or numbness.
- Immobilize the extremity with an arm board.
- Fast flush for no more than 1 second at a time to avoid sending a fluid embolus through the artery.

To protect against the risk of infection,

- Ensure that dead-end caps are securely positioned on ports.
- Change dressing using sterile technique according to institution guidelines.
- Monitor the insertion site for early signs and symptoms of infection.
- Use disposable transducers.

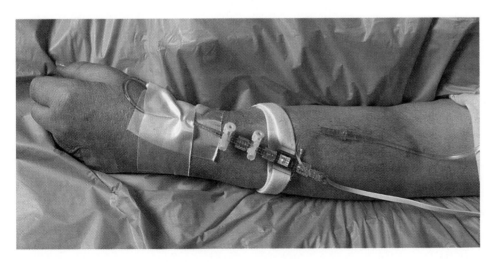

Figure 6.50 Patient with a dressed arterial line.

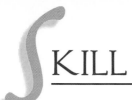

SKILL

Changing an Arterial Line Dressing

Purpose Caregivers need to be able to change an arterial line dressing whenever the dressing becomes nonocclusive, moist, or soiled. Institutional policy will also influence when a dressing is changed.

Objectives

The caregiver demonstrates the ability to do the following:

1. Gather the correct supplies.

2. Communicate using a style that reduces the patient's anxiety.

3. Maintain sterile technique.

4. Change an arterial line dressing.

5. Report the results of the procedure to the RN or preceptor.

Key Terms

Fluid-Filled Pressure Tubing Specialized rigid tubing that connects the vascular system (the artery) and the transducer.

Heparinized Solution A solution containing the drug heparin, which is used to keep the system patent.

Intraflow Device A device that limits the amount of continuous flow being delivered through the pressurized system yet allows the caregiver to flush the system after blood draws to keep it clear.

Pressure Bag A device that holds the heparinized solution under 300 mmHg pressure to maintain flow against the patient's own arterial pressure.

Transducer A device that can convert pulse waves into electrical energy that is visible on a monitor as a waveform and a systolic and diastolic number.

Supplies/ Equipment

Blue pad • Mask • Clean gloves • 2×2s • Betadine pledgets • Sterile gloves • Tape (1½″ and 1″)

Pertinent Point

When a dressing is removed, the site must be examined for signs of infection (redness, swelling, or pus). If evident, notify the physician, discontinue the arterial line, and culture the catheter tip.

Age-Specific Considerations

Older adults and patients with skin sensitivities should be monitored for skin rash or irritation. An arm board might provide greater support to the limb.

Key Concept

*A*rterial line dressing changes are routinely performed according to facility guidelines and whenever the dressing becomes nonocclusive, moist, or soiled.

1. Wash hands.

2. Identify the correct patient.

3. Explain the procedure to the patient.

4. Assemble the equipment (Figure 6.51a).

5. Place the blue pad under the patient's arm (or groin if the catheter is in the femoral artery).

6. Put on mask and clean gloves (Figure 6.51b).

7. Remove and discard the old dressing, being careful not to dislodge the catheter (Figure 6.51c).

8. Remove and discard gloves and wash hands.

9. Drop 2×2s and betadine pledgets on a sterile field.

10. Put on sterile gloves.

11. Check the site for signs of infection and irritation. (Report findings to the RN.)

12. Clean the insertion site in a circular motion with a betadine pledget; repeat (Figure 6.51d). Allow the betadine to dry.

13. Secure the tubing to the skin with tape; cover with 2×2s and additional tape (Figure 6.51e).

14. Write the date and time and your initials on the dressing (Figure 6.51f).

15. Remove and discard gloves; wash hands.

16. Document and report the results to the RN or preceptor.

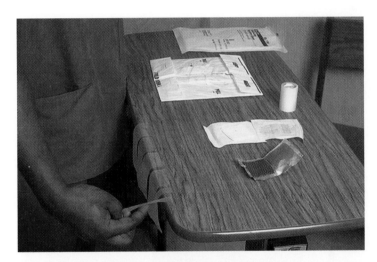

a

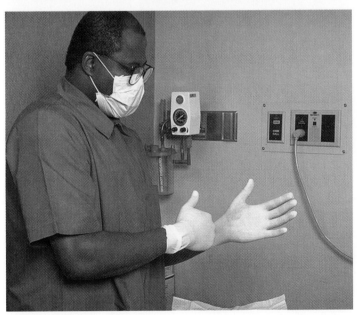

b   **Figure 6.51** Assembling the equipment.

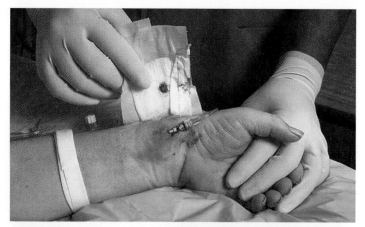

c

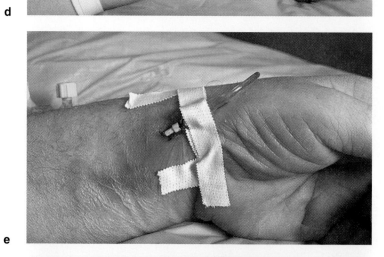

d

e

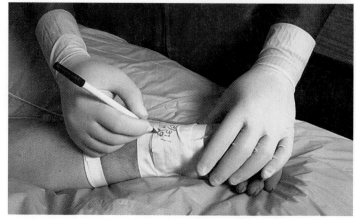

f

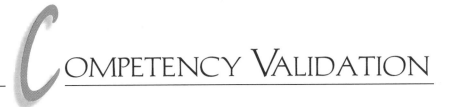

COMPETENCY VALIDATION

Skill: Changing an Arterial Line Dressing

Name _____

Preceptor _____

Date _____

Competency Statement Changes an arterial line dressing while demonstrating correct sterile technique.

Not Comeptent: _____ 1. Is <u>unable to state reason</u> for task and <u>needs instructions</u> to perform task.

_____ 2. Understands reason for task but <u>needs instructions</u> to perform task.

Competent: _____ 3. Understands reason for task and is able to perform but <u>needs to increase speed.</u>

_____ 4. Understands reason for task and is able to perform task <u>proficiently.</u>

Performance Criteria

The caregiver demonstrates the ability to do the following:

_____ 1. Wash hands.

_____ 2. Identify the correct patient.

_____ 3. Explain the procedure to the patient.

_____ 4. Assemble the equipment.

_____ a. 2x2s   _____ e. Clean gloves
_____ b. Betadine pledgets   _____ f. Mask
_____ c. Tape (½", 1")   _____ g. Blue pad
_____ d. Sterile gloves

_____ 5. Place the blue pad under the patient's arm (or groin if the catheter is in the femoral artery).

_____ 6. Put on mask and clean gloves.

_____ 7. Remove and discard the old dressing, being careful not to dislodge the catheter.

_____ 8. Remove and discard gloves; wash hands.

_____ 9. Drop 2×2s and betadine pledgets on a sterile field.

_____ 10. Put on sterile gloves.

_____ 11. Check the site for signs of infection and irritation. (Report findings to the RN.)

_____ 12. Clean the insertion site in a circular motion with a betadine pledget; repeat. Allow the betadine to dry.

_____ 13. Secure the tubing to the skin with tape; cover with 2×2s and additional tape.

_____ 14. Write the date and time and your initials on the dressing.

_____ 15. Remove and discard gloves; wash hands.

_____ 16. Document and report the results of the procedure to the RN or preceptor.

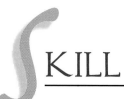

SKILL

Withdrawing Blood from an Arterial Line

Purpose Arterial lines allow convenient access to obtain frequently ordered blood specimens from unstable cardiac patients. The caregiver obtains blood samples from the arterial line stopcock port. The blood can be collected with a vacutainer or a syringe.

Objectives

The caregiver demonstrates the ability to do the following:

1. Gather the correct supplies.

2. Communicate using a style that reduces the patient's anxiety.

3. Maintain sterile technique.

4. Obtain an arterial line blood sample.

5. Report the results of the procedure to the RN or preceptor.

Key Terms

Transducer A device that can convert pulse waves into electrical energy that is visible on a monitor as a waveform and a systolic and diastolic number.

Fluid-Filled Pressure Tubing Specialized rigid tubing that connects the vascular system (the artery) and the transducer.

Heparinized Solution A solution containing the drug heparin, which is used to keep the system patent.

Pressure Bag A device that holds the heparinized solution under 300 mmHg pressure to maintain flow against the patient's own arterial pressure.

Intraflow Device A device that limits the amount of continuous flow being delivered through the pressurized system yet allows the caregiver to flush the system after blood draws to keep it clear.

Supplies/ Equipment

Clean gloves • Lab slips stamped with patient name, date, time, and unit phone number • Blood tubes and/or heparinized syringe for specimens • Alcohol wipes • Vacutainer holder with protected needle adapter or syringe • Syringe or red-top tube for discard • 2×2 or medicine cup • Plastic bag • Ice, if drawing blood gas specimens

Pertinent Point

Arterial blood gas specimens must be transported to the lab on ice to obtain valid results.

The portion of blood that is mixed with the heparinized saline solution must not be used or sent as the test sample. Discard 3 cc of blood for all tests, unless drawing coagulation studies.

If drawing numerous tests with coagulation studies, at least 10 cc of blood must be obtained before drawing the coagulation studies. If coags are the only tests needed, use a 10-cc red-top for the discard tube, then proceed with drawing the coagulation studies.

Put the blood sample into labeled tubes. For multiple tubes, fill red (or yellow) first, then blue, and then purple.

1. Wash hands.
2. Identify the correct patient.
3. Explain the procedure to the patient.
4. Assemble the equipment, and apply gloves.
5. Label the appropriate tubes with patient name, date, time, and unit phone number.
6. Suspend the monitor alarm.
7. Remove the Luer Lok cap from the distal stopcock, and maintain sterility (Figure 6.52a).
8. Wipe the open end of the stopcock with an alcohol wipe, and allow to dry (Figure 6.52b).
9. Perform the procedure for a vacutainer blood draw:
   a. Attach the adapter and the vacutainer to the stopcock. Then place an unlabeled discard tube over the needle, and open the stopcock to the vacutainer.
   b. Discard 3 cc of blood for all tests, unless drawing coagulation studies. If drawing numerous tests with coagulation studies, obtain at least 10 cc of blood before drawing the coagulation studies. If coags are the only tests needed, use a 10-cc red-top for the discard tube, then proceed with drawing the coagulation studies.

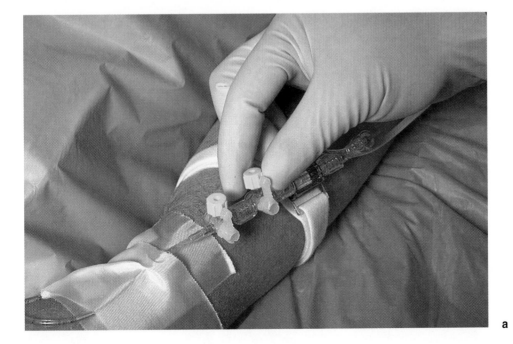

Figure 6.52
Removing the cap from the distal stopcock on a four-way or Luer Lok stopcock.

a

c. Put the blood sample into the labeled tubes. For multiple tubes, fill red (or yellow) first, then blue, and then purple.

d. Close the stopcock to the patient. Remove the vacutainer. Flush out the stopcock into a 2×2 or medicine cup.

e. Close the stopcock to the atmosphere.

f. Replace the dead-end cap.

g. Flush the patient line in short, one-second increments, until it is clear of blood.

h. Turn the monitor alarm back on.

i. Place blood specimens in a plastic bag.

j. Dispose of equipment.

k. Wash hands thoroughly.

l. Document on nursing flowsheet—or patient record—time blood was drawn and what specimen(s) were sent to lab.

10. Perform the procedure for a syringe blood draw:

a. Suspend the arterial line alarm.

b. Attach the discard syringe to the stopcock, and open the stopcock to the syringe (Figure 6.52c).

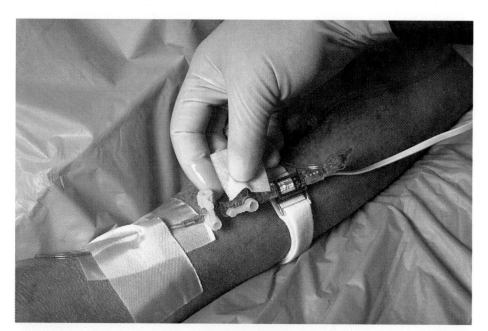

b

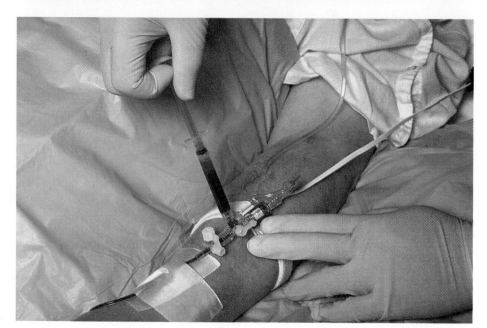

c

c. Discard 3 cc of blood for all tests, unless drawing coagulation studies. If drawing numerous tests with coagulation studies, obtain at least 10 cc of blood before drawing the coagulation studies. If coags are the only tests needed, use a 10-cc red-top for the discard tube, then proceed with drawing the coagulation studies.

d. Turn the stopcock to a 45-degree angle. Then remove the syringe (Figure 6.52d).

e. Attach the sample syringe, and open the stopcock to withdraw the blood sample (Figure 6.52e). Be careful of accidental disconnection with non–Leur Lok syringes. Repeat as necessary, closing the stopcock to a 45-degree angle between syringe changes.

f. Close the stopcock to the patient, and flush out the stopcock into a 2×2 or medicine cup (Figure 6.52f).

g. Close the stopcock to the atmosphere. Apply the dead-endercap.

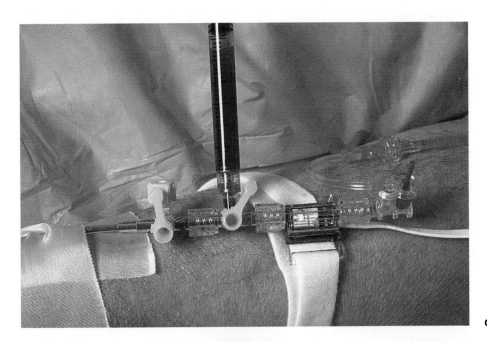

d

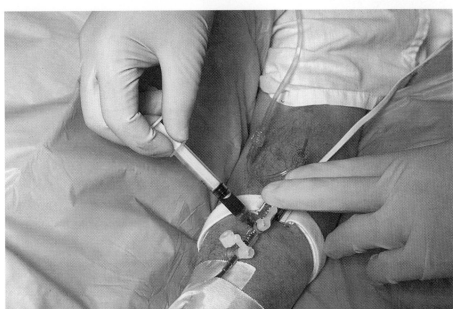

e

h. Replace the dead-end cap (Figure 6.52g).

i. Flush the patient line in short, one-second increments, until it is clear of blood (Figure 6.52h).

j. Turn the monitor alarm back on.

k. Transfer blood from the syringes into labeled tubes.

l. Place blood specimens in a plastic bag.

m. Dispose of equipment (Figure 6.52i).

11. Remove and discard gloves; wash hands.

12. Document on the nursing flow sheet what time the blood was drawn and what specimens were sent to the lab.

13. Report the results to the RN or preceptor.

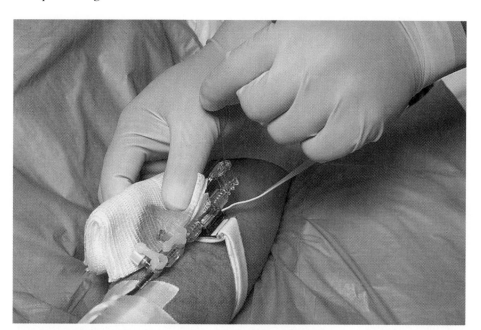

f

g

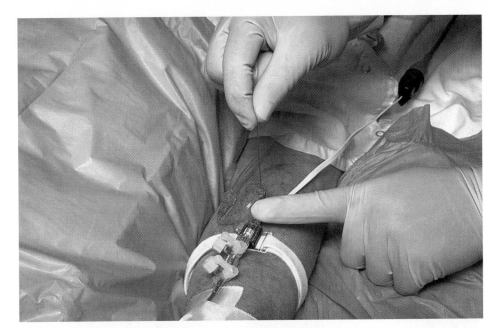

h

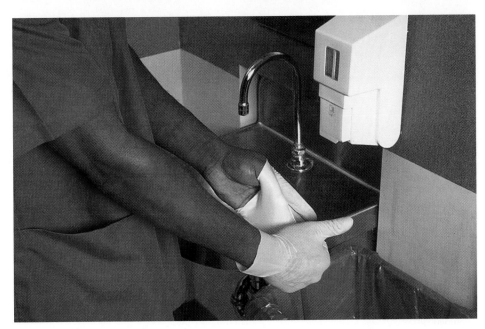

i

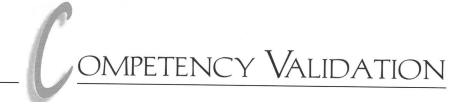

COMPETENCY VALIDATION

Skill: Withdrawing Blood from an Arterial Line

Name _____

Preceptor _____

Date _____

Competency Statement Withdraws blood from an arterial line while demonstrating correct sterile technique.

Not Competent:

_____ 1. Is <u>unable to state reason</u> for task and <u>needs instructions</u> to perform task.

_____ 2. Understands reason for task but <u>needs instructions</u> to perform task.

Competent:

_____ 3. Understands reason for task and is able to perform task but <u>needs to increase speed.</u>

_____ 4. Understands reason for task and is able to perform task <u>proficiently.</u>

Performance Criteria

The caregiver demonstrates the ability to do the following:

_____ 1. Wash hands.

_____ 2. Identify the correct patient.

_____ 3. Explain the procedure to the patient.

_____ 4. Assemble the equipment, and apply gloves.

　　_____ a. Alcohol wipes.

　　_____ b. 2×2 or medicine cup.

　　_____ c. Ice, if drawing blood gases.

　　_____ d. Plastic bag.

_____ 5. Label the appropriate tubes.

_____ 6. Suspend the monitor alarm.

_____ 7. Remove the Luer Lok cap from the distal stopcock, and maintain sterility.

_____ 8. Wipe the open end of the stopcock with an alcohol wipe, and allow to dry.

_____ 9. Perform the procedure for a vacutainer blood draw:

　　_____ a. Attach the adapter and the vacutainer to the stopcock. Then place an unlabeled discard tube over the needle, and open the stopcock to the vacutainer.

　　_____ b. Discard 3 cc of blood for all tests, unless drawing coagulation studies. If drawing numerous tests with coagulation studies, obtain at least 10 cc of blood before drawing the coagulation studies. If coags are the only tests needed, use a 10-cc red-top for the discard tube, then proceed with drawing the coagulation studies.

　　_____ c. Obtain the blood sample into the labeled tubes. For multiple tubes, fill red (or yellow) first, then blue, and then purple.

　　_____ d. Close the stopcock to the patient. Remove the vacutainer. Flush out the stopcock into a 2×2 or medicine cup.

　　_____ e. Close the stopcock to the atmosphere.

　　_____ f. Replace the dead-end cap.

　　_____ g. Flush the patient line in short, one-second increments, until it is clear of blood.

　　_____ h. Turn the monitor alarm back on.

　　_____ i. Place blood specimens in a plastic bag.

　　_____ j. Dispose of equipment.

　　_____ k. Wash hands thoroughly.

　　_____ l. Document on nursing flow sheet—or patient record—time blood drawn and what specimen(s) were sent to lab.

_____ 10. Perform the procedure for a syringe blood draw:

　　_____ a. Suspend the arterial line alarm.

　　_____ b. Attach the discard syringe to the stopcock, and open the stopcock to the syringe.

　　_____ c. Discard 3 cc of blood for all tests, unless drawing coagulation studies. If drawing numerous tests with coagulation studies, obtain at least 10 cc of blood before drawing the coagulation studies. If coags are the only tests needed, use a 10-cc red-top for the discard tube, then proceed with drawing the coagulation studies.

　　_____ d. Turn the stopcock to a 45-degree angle. Then remove the syringe, and draw the blood specimens for the lab.

　　_____ e. Attach the sample syringe, and open the stopcock to withdraw the blood sample. Be careful of accidental disconnection with non–Leur Lok syringes. Repeat as necessary, closing the stopcock to a 45-degree angle between syringe changes.

　　_____ f. Close the stopcock to the patient, and flush out the stopcock into a 2×2 or medicine cup.

　　_____ g. Close the stopcock to the atmosphere.

　　_____ h. Replace the dead-end cap.

　　_____ i. Flush the patient line in short, one-second increments, until it is clear of blood.

　　_____ j. Turn the monitor alarm back on.

　　_____ k. Transfer blood from the syringes into labeled tubes.

　　_____ l. Place blood specimens in a plastic bag.

　　_____ m. Dispose of equipment.

_____ 11. Remove and discard gloves; wash hands.

_____ 12. Document on the nursing flow sheet what time the blood was drawn and what specimens were sent to the lab.

_____ 13. Report the results to the RN or preceptor.

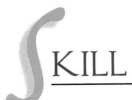

SKILL

Removing an Arterial Line

Purpose Caregivers remove arterial lines when the patient no longer requires one or when there is evidence of an infection.

The caregiver demonstrates the ability to do the following:

Objectives

1. Gather the correct supplies.
2. Communicate using a style that reduces the patient's anxiety.
3. Maintain sterile technique.
4. Correctly remove an arterial line catheter and apply a pressure dressing.
5. Respond appropriately to possible complications.
6. Report the results of the procedure to the RN or preceptor.

Key Terms

Transducer A device that can convert pulse waves into electrical energy that is visible on a monitor as a waveform and a systolic and diastolic number.

Fluid-filled Pressure Tubing Specialized rigid tubing that connects the vascular system (the artery) and the transducer.

Heparinized Solution A solution containing the drug heparin, which is used to keep the system patent.

Pressure Bag A device that holds the heparinized solution under 300 mmHg pressure to maintain flow against the patient's own arterial pressure.

Intraflow Device A device that limits the amount of continuous flow being delivered through the pressurized system yet allows the caregiver to flush the system after blood draws to keep it clear.

Supplies/ Equipment

Blue pad • Clean gloves • Sterile gloves • Suture removal kit • Sterile 4×4s • Tape

Pertinent Point

The discontinuation of an arterial line requires sterile technique.

Age-Specific Considerations

Older adults or those patients with very sensitive or fragile skin might benefit from hyperallergenic or paper tape to secure their dressing. The dressing is applied after the arterial line is removed.

Key Concept

*F*irm pressure must be maintained over the site for at least 5 minutes for radial catheters and at least 10 minutes for femoral catheters until bleeding has completely stopped. Uncontrolled arterial bleeding can result in death.

$Steps$

1. Wash hands.
2. Identify the correct patient.
3. Explain the procedure to the patient.
4. Assemble the equipment.
5. Turn the arterial line monitor alarm off.
6. Place the blue pad under the patient's arm (or groin if the catheter is in the femoral artery).

7. Close the arterial catheter stopcock to the patient (Figure 6.53a).
8. Deflate the pressure bag (Figure 6.53b).
9. Put on clean gloves.
10. Remove and discard the arterial line dressing, being careful not to dislodge the catheter.
11. Remove and discard gloves; wash hands.
12. Put on sterile gloves.

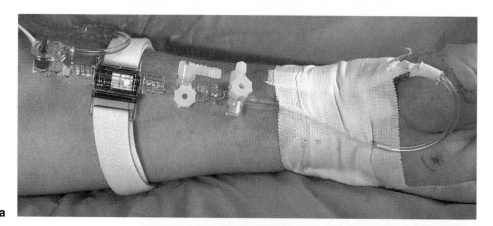

Figure 6.53
Removing an arterial line.

a

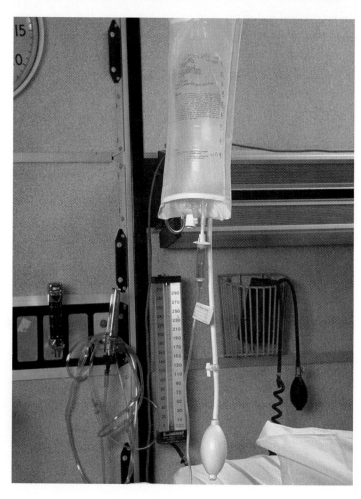

b

13. Cut and remove the skin sutures while stabilizing the catheter (Figure 6.53c).

14. Withdraw the catheter, and immediately apply firm pressure directly over the site with a 4×4 (Figure 6.53d).

15. Stand by as the RN assesses the integrity of the catheter and documents the condition of the site and the time of removal.

16. Place fingertips of one hand over the artery, and apply firm pressure for a minimum of 5 minutes for radial sites and 10 minutes for femoral sites.

17. Check the site; if bleeding or sudden swelling occurs, reapply firm pressure for an additional 5 to 10 minutes; continue until bleeding stops.

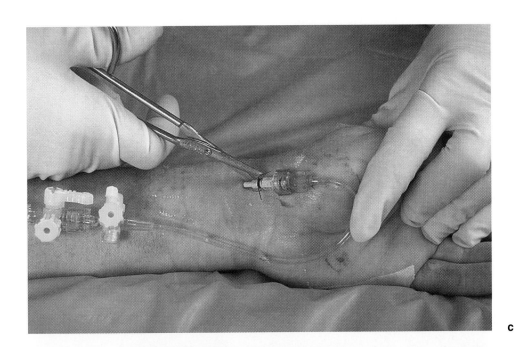

c

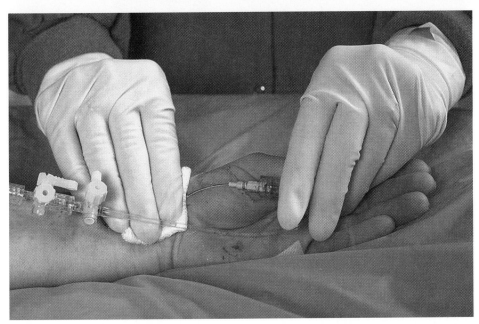

d

18. After the RN checks the site, place one sterile folded 4×4 (or 2×2s) over the puncture site, and tape firmly to apply pressure (Figure 6.53e).

19. Write the date and time and your initials on the pressure dressing.

20. Instruct the patient to avoid putting pressure on the affected extremity for a few hours and to notify the staff if the dressing feels warm or wet. Reapply pressure immediately for bleeding or sudden swelling. The pressure dressing may be removed after 8 hours.

21. Disconnect and discard the tubing, and empty the infusion bag into the sink.

22. Do not discard the cable or the pressure bag.

23. Dispose of the suture removal kit and any sharps in the sharps container.

24. Return the cable and the pressure bag to the appropriate place on the unit.

25. Notify the RN of any bleeding, swelling, ecchymosis, complaints of pain, or numbness.

26. Document and report the results to the RN or preceptor.

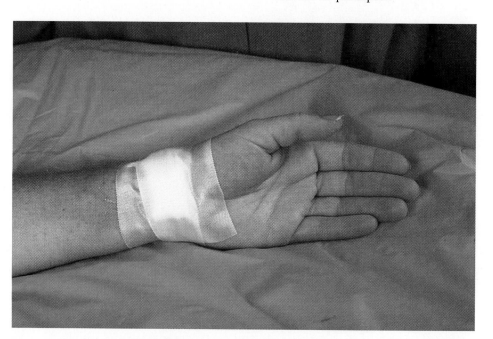

e

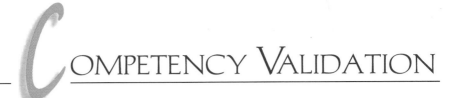

COMPETENCY VALIDATION

Skill: Removing an Arterial Line

Name _____

Preceptor _____

Date _____

Competency Statement Removes an arterial line while demonstrating correct sterile technique.

Not Competent: _____ 1. Is <u>unable to state reason</u> for task and <u>needs instructions</u> to perform task.

_____ 2. Understands reason for task but <u>needs instructions</u> to perform task.

Competent: _____ 3. Understands reason for task and is able to perform task but <u>needs to increase speed.</u>

_____ 4. Understands reason for task and is able to perform task <u>proficiently.</u>

Performance Criteria

The caregiver demonstrates the ability to do the following:

_____ 1. Wash hands.

_____ 2. Identify the correct patient.

_____ 3. Explain the procedure to the patient.

_____ 4. Assemble the equipment.

_____ 5. Turn the arterial line monitor alarm off.

_____ 6. Place the blue pad under the patient's arm (or groin if the catheter is in the femoral artery).

_____ 7. Close the arterial catheter stopcock to the patient.

_____ 8. Deflate the pressure bag.

_____ 9. Put on clean gloves.

_____ 10. Remove and discard the arterial line dressing, being careful not to dislodge the catheter.

_____ 11. Remove and discard gloves.

_____ 12. Put on sterile gloves.

_____ 13. Cut and remove the skin sutures while stabilizing the catheter.

_____ 14. Withdraw the catheter, and immediately apply firm pressure directly over the side with a 4×4.

_____ 15. Stand by as the RN assesses the integrity of the catheter and documents the condition of the site and the time of removal.

_____ 16. Place fingertips of one hand over the artery, and apply firm pressure for a minimum of 5 minutes for radial sites and 10 minutes for femoral sites.

_____ 17. Check the site; if bleeding or sudden swelling occurs, reapply firm pressure for an additional 5 to 10 minutes; continue until bleeding stops.

_____ 18. After the RN checks the site, place one sterile folded 4×4 (or 2×2s) over the puncture site, and tape firmly to apply pressure.

_____ 19. Write the date and time and your initials on the pressure dressing.

_____ 20. Instruct the patient to avoid putting pressure on the affected extremity for a few hours and to notify the staff if the dressing feels warm or wet. Reapply pressure immediately for bleeding or sudden swelling. The pressure dressing may be removed after 8 hours.

_____ 21. Disconnect and discard the tubing, and empty the infusion bag into the sink.

_____ 22. Do not discard the cable or pressure bag.

_____ 23. Dispose of the suture removal kit and any sharps in the sharps container.

_____ 24. Return the cable and the pressure bag to the appropriate place on the unit.

_____ 25. Notify the RN of any bleeding, swelling, ecchymosis, complaints of pain, or numbness.

_____ 26. Document and report the results to the RN or preceptor.

SKILL

Palpating Dorsalis Pedis and Posterior Tibial Pulses

Purpose The purpose of palpating the dorsalis pedis and posterior tibial pulses is to check the flow of blood or the presence of blood circulation to the feet and toes (Figure 6.54). This is very important when caring for patients with circulation disorders or patients who have had procedures that assess the status of their circulation. These pulses are located and assessed before and after the patient has the procedure.

Objectives

The caregiver demonstrates the ability to do the following:

1. Gather the correct supplies.

2. Communicate using a style that reduces the patient's anxiety.

3. Correctly identify the presence of the dorsalis pedis and posterior tibial pulses.

4. Report the results of the procedure to the RN or preceptor.

Key Terms

Doppler The machine that locates pulses based on the Doppler effect. There is a change in the frequency of sound waves as the probe (sensor) gets closer to the pulse of the patient. The sound decreases as the probe gets farther away from the pulse.

Dorsalis Pedis (DP) Pulse The pulse of the dorsalis pedis artery, which supplies blood to various muscles of the foot and toes. In about 90 percent of people, it is located between the first and second toes on the top of the foot.

Posterior Tibial (PT) Pulse The pulse of the posterior tibial artery, which supplies blood to a variety of muscles in the lower leg, foot, and toes. It is located in the inner aspect of the ankle, just below the anklebone.

Supplies/
Equipment

Doppler machine • Doppler jelly • Marker • Washcloth

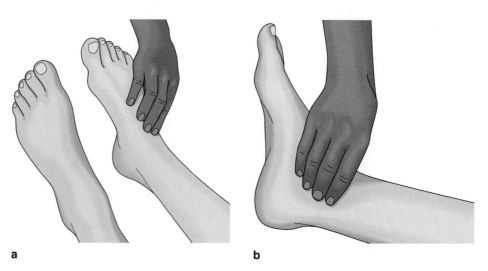

a   b

Figure 6.54 Checking (a) dorsalis pedis pulse and (b) posterior tibial pulse.

- The DP and PT pulses can be palpated using your index and middle fingers.
- Because of chronic medical conditions—such as atherosclerosis, diabetes, and peripheral vascular disease—a patient's pulses might be very weak or impossible to palpate. In this case, a Doppler machine is used to obtain the pulses.
- Signs of reduced or poor circulation are skin that blanches slowly, skin that is very pale or dusky, and even necrotic areas on the lower legs, toes, or feet.
- The sudden absence of the DP or PT pulse after a procedure signals that an occlusion has occurred in the peripheral circulation. This is a medical emergency and requires immediate action. Notify the RN immediately. The RN will inform the physician of the patient's loss of the pulse, vital signs, and general condition.

Due to hereditary and lifestyle factors, as people age they sometimes become more susceptible to chronic diseases that reduce the amount of blood flow throughout the body. The skin on their feet might be very fragile or thick and tough. Some people are sensitive to the coldness of the Doppler jelly. Out of respect for the seriousness of these conditions, do not rush patients. Give them time to ask questions. Be respectful at all times, and acknowledge the anxiety that is a part of all of these procedures. Inform all patients of what you are doing and why. Keep the patient's feet covered with blankets between pulse checks.

*T*he presence of the pulses indicates that an occlusion has not formed and that the circulation to the feet and toes is intact. If a pulse is lost (cannot be palpated), there has been a blockage of the circulation, often due to a blood clot.

1. Wash hands.
2. Identify the correct patient.
3. Explain the procedure to the patient.
4. Assemble the equipment.
5. Uncover the patient's feet by untucking the sheets at the end of the bed. Leave the covers over the patient's body for warmth and privacy.
6. With a gentle but firm touch (avoid tickling), feel for the DP pulse (on the top of the patient's foot, between the first and second toes). If you are unable to palpate any pulse after trying for several minutes, use a Doppler machine:

a. Apply the Doppler jelly to the area where the DP pulse should be located.
b. Apply the Doppler pencil or sensor on the jelly. Slowly move the sensor until the pulse is audible. Listen for a whooshing sound.
c. Using the marker, note the location of the pulse with an *X* on the patient's skin (Figure 6.55a). This will help with the next pulse check (Figure 6.55b).
d. Wipe off the excess Doppler jelly with the washcloth.

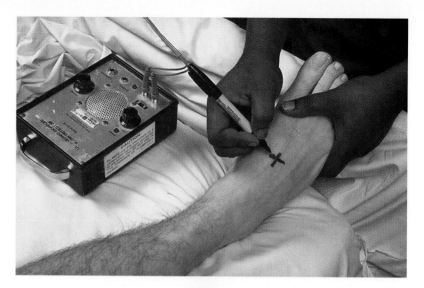

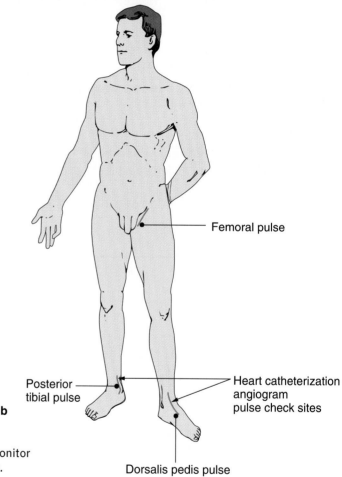

Femoral pulse

Posterior tibial pulse

Heart catheterization angiogram pulse check sites

Dorsalis pedis pulse

a

b

Figure 6.55 (a) Marking a pulse. (b) Pulse sites to monitor during a post-heart catheterization/angiogram check.

7. Using the same gentle but firm touch, palpate the PT pulse (inner aspect of the ankle below the ankle-bone). You might need to use the Doppler again to locate the pulse.

8. Mark the location of the PT pulse with the marker on the patient's skin.

9. Turn off the Doppler. Cover the patient's feet for warmth.

10. Document the presence of the pulses by indicating whether each was positive (+) or negative (−).

11. Report the results to the RN or preceptor.

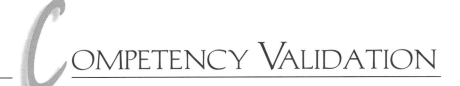

COMPETENCY VALIDATION

Skill: Palpating Dorsalis Pedis and Posterior Tibial Pulses

Name _____

Preceptor _____

Date _____

Competency Statement Palpates dorsalis pedis and posterior tibial pulses while demonstrating correct technique.

Not Competent: _____ 1. Is <u>unable to state reason</u> for task and <u>needs instructions</u> to perform task.

_____ 2. Understands reason for task but <u>needs instructions</u> to perform task.

Competent: _____ 3. Understands reason for task and is able to perform task but <u>needs to increase speed.</u>

_____ 4. Understands reason for task and is able to perform task <u>proficiently.</u>

Performance Criteria

The caregiver demonstrates the ability to do the following:

_____ 1. Wash hands.

_____ 2. Identify the correct patient.

_____ 3. Explain the procedure to the patient.

_____ 4. Assemble the equipment.

_____ 5. Uncover the patient's feet by untucking the sheets at the end of the bed. Leave the covers over the patient's body for warmth and privacy.

_____ 6. With a gentle but firm touch (avoid tickling), feel for the DP pulse (on the top of the patient's foot, between the first and second toes). If you are unable to palpate any pulse after trying for several minutes, use a Doppler machine:

a. Apply the Doppler jelly to the area where the DP pulse should be located.

b. Apply the Doppler pencil or sensor on the jelly. Slowly move the sensor until the pulse is audible. Listen for a whooshing sound.

c. Using the marker, note the location of the pulse with an *X* on the patient's skin. This will help with the next pulse check.

d. Wipe off the excess Doppler jelly with the washcloth.

_____ 7. Using the same gentle but firm touch, palpate the PT pulse (inner aspect of the ankle below the anklebone). You might need to use the Doppler again to locate the pulse.

_____ 8. Mark the location of the PT pulse with the marker on the patient's skin.

_____ 9. Turn off the Doppler. Cover the patient's feet for warmth.

_____ 10. Document the presence of the pulses by indicating whether each was positive (+) or negative (−).

_____ 11. Report the results to the RN or preceptor.

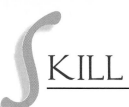

SKILL

Removing a PTCA Femoral Sheath

Purpose Percutaneous transluminal coronary angioplasty (PTCA) has been used with increasing frequency to treat patients with coronary artery disease. Many cardiac patients are sent to intermediate or progressive care units with femoral sheaths in place. Before RNs or patient care technicians (PCTs) can discontinue these lines, caregivers must demonstrate competency in manual compression and in the use of the C-clamp, which is a mechanical compression device (Figure 6.56).

Objectives

The caregiver demonstrates the ability to do the following:

1. Gather the correct supplies.

2. Communicate using a style that reduces the patient's anxiety.

3. Remove a femoral sheath using manual compression.

4. Remove a femoral sheath using a C-clamp.

5. Describe possible complications associated with the procedure.

6. Report the results of the procedure to the RN or preceptor.

Key Terms

C-clamp A mechanical device that holds pressure on a blood vessel.

Femoral Sheath A large catheter placed in the femoral artery that provides an entryway so that the balloon angioplasty catheter can be placed and threaded to the coronary arteries. The sheath is left in after removal of the angioplasty catheter until coagulation studies are near normal. The sheath is then removed.

Hemostasis The formation of a blood clot.

Hematoma A mass that forms when blood escapes the vessel and goes out into the tissues or a cavity. Bruising usually results.

Manual Compression A technique in which the caregiver uses the hands to compress a blood vessel to stop the bleeding.

Vasovagal Response A response that can occur when the vagus nerve is stimulated during compression of the femoral artery. Symptoms include a decrease in the level of consciousness; cold, clammy skin; pale skin; nausea and vomiting; decreased blood pressure; and a decrease in the heart rate.

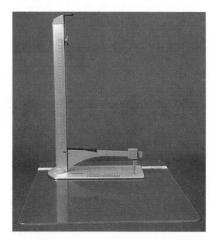

Figure 6.56 Plexiglas board and C-clamp.

Doppler machine • Doppler jelly • Tape • Clean gloves • Sterile gloves • Suture removal kit • Sterile 4×4s • Plexiglas board, C-clamp, and sterile disc (if appropriate) • Butterfly dressing • Personal protective equipment: apron and goggles

- Since percutaneous transluminal coronary angioplasty was first introduced in 1977, it has been used with increasing frequency to treat patients with coronary artery disease. It is estimated that more than five hundred thousand angioplasties are performed in the United States annually.

- PTCA is a nonsurgical procedure that uses a balloon to dilate the diseased coronary arteries. The balloon catheter is advanced through a larger sheath in the femoral artery. The sheath provides structural support in the artery for the catheters used in the procedure. After the PTCA, the sheath is left in place from 4 to 12 hours to allow easy access for restudy if needed. Some sheaths are removed as soon as a coagulation study—for example, an automated coagulation timer (ACT) or partial thromboplastin time (PTT)—is within a safe range to avoid bleeding complications.

- While still in place, the sheath may be used as an arterial line to draw blood for lab tests. The sheath is connected to a pressurized bag of normal saline with heparin—the same one used for radial arterial lines to maintain patency of the line. A number of different-size sheaths are made by different manufacturers. Before drawing blood to be sent to the lab, discard approximately three times the amount of dead space of the sheath (approximately 5 cc for a size 7 or 8 French). The stopcock closest to the patient can be used. For coagulation studies, six times the dead space (or approximately 10 cc) is discarded before drawing the specimen. Check the manufacturer's recommendations for the catheters used in your facility.

- Most angioplasty patients can have the sheath removed using pressure for approximately 15 to 30 minutes. In patients with an intracoronary stent (a metal device that is implanted to hold the artery open), the compression time increases from 30 to 60 minutes, depending on institution protocol. Generally, these patients receive more medications to thin the blood, causing more risk for bleeding—thus the longer compression time.

- Complications associated with this procedure include hematoma (swelling or massing of blood into the surrounding tissues), inadequate blood flow to the foot, bleeding, and vasovagal response. A vasovagal response includes any of the following symptoms: decreased level of consciousness; cold, clammy, pale skin; nausea and vomiting; decrease in blood pressure; and decrease in heart rate.

- When using the manual method, the caregiver must maintain straight wrist alignment while using either two fingers or two knuckles to apply pressure on the femoral pulse above the site.

Fewer premedication narcotics might be required before a sheath removal in an older adult due to the metabolism of these drugs in older patients. Care should be taken when lifting the C-clamp disc, as it might stick to fragile skin and cause a break in the skin. Gently break the suction of the disc against the skin, using the fingertip, before removal.

*A*n RN must be present during a sheath removal to manage the patient in case he or she experiences a vasovagal response while another RN or caregiver removes the sheath. The RN must remain in the patient's room during and for at least 5 minutes after the procedure. The RN will give the patient sedation as ordered. Atropine (a medication that can increase the heart rate) can be given intravenously by the RN, along with a fluid bolus, according to established protocols.

Steps

1. Perform the procedure only after being instructed to do so by the RN. (The RN must identify whether the patient's ACT or PTT results indicate readiness to have the sheath removed.)

2. Wash hands.

3. Identify the correct patient.

4. Explain the procedure to the patient.

5. Assemble the equipment, and inform the RN when ready to perform the procedure (Figures 6.57a and b).

6. Locate the dorsalis pedis pulse, and secure the Doppler in place with tape (Figure 6.57c).

7. Adjust the height of the bed so that your body can be positioned directly over the patient. Place the nurse call light within easy reach.

8. Wash hands thoroughly. Put on clean gloves and personal protective equipment (apron and goggles).

9. Remove the dressing from the groin. Discard the dressing and gloves; wash hands.

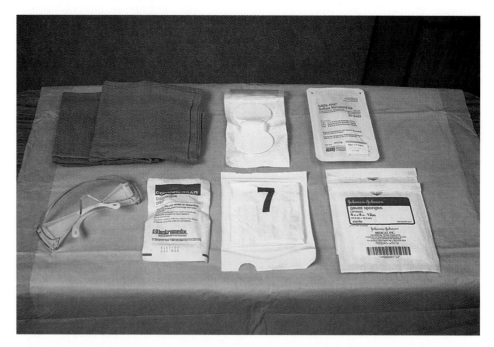

Figure 6.57a Assemble supplies and equipment including Plexiglas board and C-clamp (see Figure 6.57b).

10. Put on sterile gloves, and remove sutures from around the sheath site (Figure 6.57d).

11. Instruct the patient to breathe normally during sheath removal to avoid decreased heart rate due to vasovagal response.

12. Locate the femoral pulse.

13. Remove the sheath:
    a. Visualize the site.
    b. Use a single layer of gauze.
    c. Apply firm, focused pressure.

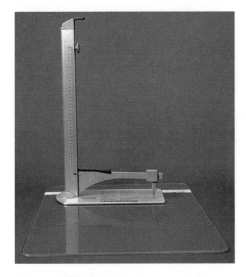

Figure 6.57b Plexiglas board and C-clamp.

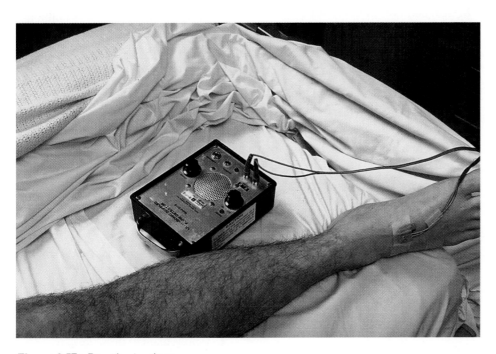

Figure 6.57c Doppler in place.

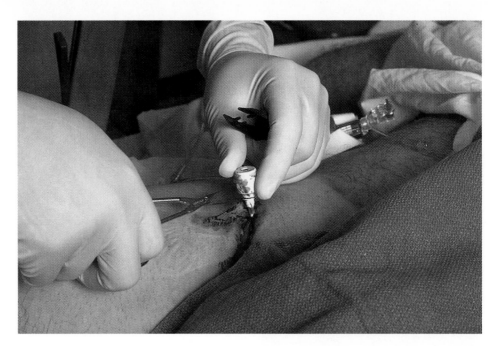

Figure 6.57d Suture removal.

d. Position hand correctly.

e. Pull the sheath in one smooth, steady motion.

14. **Manual Method:**

a. Apply firm pressure above the puncture site until hemostasis is achieved. The RN will monitor the ECG for vasovagal responses.

b. Maintain firm pressure for 15 to 20 minutes.

c. Occlude the dorsalis pedis pulse for 3 to 5 minutes. Then release just enough pressure so that you can hear a faint pulse over the Doppler.

d. Release pressure *slowly* after 15 to 20 minutes, and watch for bleeding.

e. If bleeding continues, reapply pressure for 5 to 10 minutes, then check again for continued bleeding. Continue until bleeding stops.

C-clamp Method:

a. Apply pressure using the C-clamp.

b. Position the Plexiglas board under the patient to provide a firm surface to place the C-clamp on (Figure 6.58a).

c. Position the C-clamp on the Plexiglas board but under the patient.

d. Attach the sterile disc to the tip of the compressor arm.

e. Position the C-clamp disc above the puncture site so that it can be lowered, with pressure applied, while the sheath is removed (Figures 6.58b, c, and d). Take care not to apply too much pressure before the sheath is out. This can cause a milking effect on any clot that is within the sheath.

f. Apply firm pressure above the puncture site until hemostasis is achieved. The RN will monitor the ECG for vasovagal responses.

g. Occlude the dorsalis pedis pulse for 3 to 5 minutes. Then release just enough pressure to allow some blood flow to the foot. A slight pulse will be audible over the Doppler.

h. Release the pressure *slowly,* using the release level on the C-clamp, after 15 to 20 minutes. Watch for bleeding (Figures 6.58e and f).

i. If bleeding continues, reapply the C-clamp.

j. Apply manual pressure if bleeding cannot be controlled with the C-clamp.

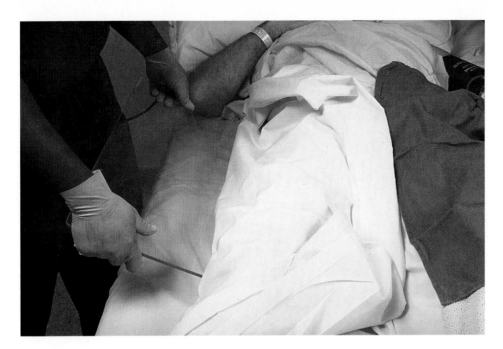

a

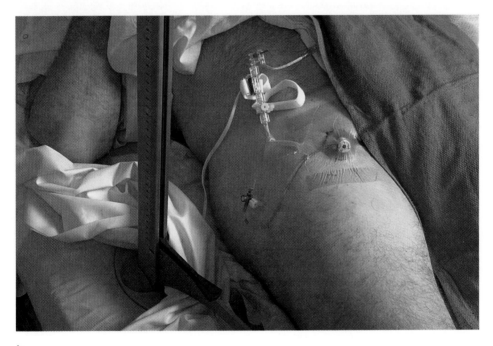

b

Figure 6.58 Positioning the C-clamp.

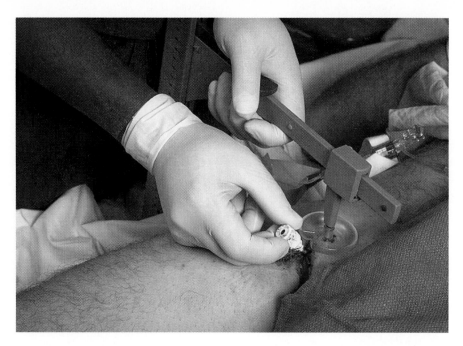

c

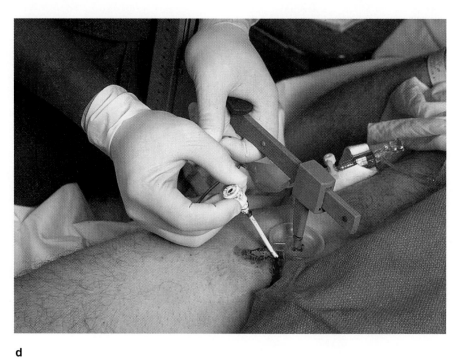

d

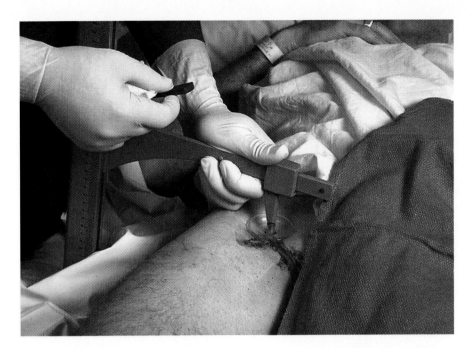

e

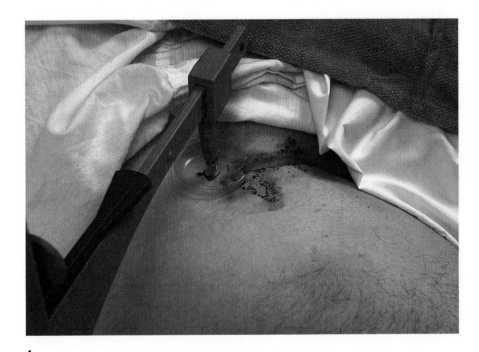

f

15. Observe the site for 3 to 5 minutes before applying the butterfly dressing (Figure 6.58g).

16. Document the patient's vital signs, pedal pulse checks, and dressing checks every 15 minutes for a half hour, then every 30 minutes for an hour, then every hour for 4 hours, and every 4 hours until patient is discharged. Check under the dressing for bleeding.

17. Notify the RN immediately if you note any of the following: abnormalities in vital signs, chest pain, bleeding on dressing, hematoma, or diminished pedal pulses.

18. Instruct the patient to call for the RN for any of the following signs:

    a. Signs of bleeding, feelings of warm blood oozing, or stickiness

    b. Signs of compromised circulation—coolness, numbness, pain, dizziness

    c. Signs of hematoma

    d. Chest pain

19. Instruct the patient to remain flat in bed (or with the head of the bed up 15 degrees), usually for 4 to 6 hours. Then the patient can be up with assistance. The patient may be logrolled.

20. Remind the patient to apply firm pressure directly on the dressing over the insertion site whenever laughing, coughing, sneezing, bearing down, or tightening the abdominal muscles in any way.

21. Discard the dressings, sheath, and gloves in the appropriate medical waste container.

22. Document and report the results to the RN or preceptor.

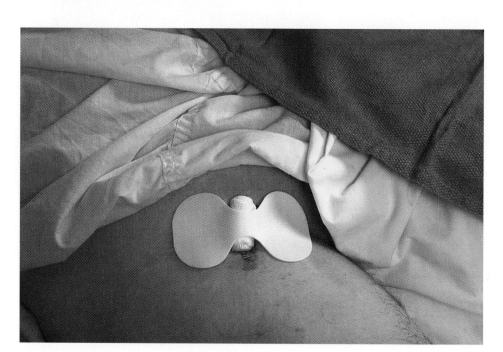

g

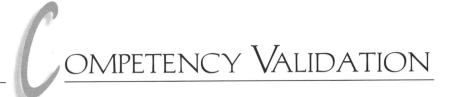

Skill: Removing a PTCA Femoral Sheath

Name _____

Preceptor _____

Date _____

Competency Statement Removes a PTCA femoral sheath while demonstrating correct sterile technique.

Not Competent: _____ 1. Is <u>unable to state reason</u> for task and <u>needs instructions</u> to perform task.

_____ 2. Understands reason for task but <u>needs instructions</u> to perform task.

Competent: _____ 3. Understands reason for task and is able to perform task but <u>needs to increase speed.</u>

_____ 4. Understands reason for task and is able to perform task <u>proficiently.</u>

Performance Criteria

The caregiver demonstrates the ability to do the following:

_____ 1. Perform the procedure only after being instructed to do so by the RN. (The RN must identify whether the patient's ACT or PTT results indicate readiness to have the sheath removed.)

_____ 2. Wash hands.

_____ 3. Identify the correct patient.

_____ 4. Explain the procedure to the patient.

_____ 5. Assemble the equipment, and inform the RN when ready to perform the procedure.

_____ a. Doppler and gel, suture removal kit, 4×4s (approx. 2), sterile gloves, clean gloves, butterfly dressing, C-clamp and sterile disc (if appropriate), Plexiglas board, personal protective equipment.

_____ b. RN *must* remain in the patient's room during and for at least 5 minutes after the PTCA sheath is removed. RN will give the patient sedation as ordered.

_____ 6. Locate the dorsalis pedis pulse, and secure the Doppler in place with tape.

_____ 7. Adjust the height of the bed so that your body can be positioned directly over the patient. Place the nurse call light within easy reach.

_____ 8. Wash hands thoroughly, and put on clean gloves.

_____ 9. Remove the dressing from the groin. Discard the dressing and gloves.

_____ 10. Put on sterile gloves, and remove sutures from around the sheath site.

_____ 11. Instruct the patient to breathe normally during sheath removal to avoid decreased heart rate due to vasovagal response.

_____ 12. Locate the femoral pulse.

_____ 13. Remove the sheath:

_____ a. Visualize the site.

_____ b. Use a single layer of gauze.

_____ c. Apply firm, focused pressure.

_____ d. Position hand correctly.

_____ e. Pull the sheath in one smooth, steady motion.

_____ 14. **Manual Method:**

        _____ a. Apply firm pressure above the puncture site until hemostasis is achieved. The RN will monitor the ECG for vasovagal responses.

        _____ b. Maintain firm pressure for 15 to 20 minutes.

        _____ c. Occlude the dorsalis pedis pulse for 3 to 5 minutes. Then release just enough pressure so that you can hear a faint pulse over the Doppler.

        _____ d. Release pressure *slowly* after 15 to 20 minutes, and watch for bleeding.

        _____ e. If bleeding continues, reapply pressure for 5 to 10 minutes, then check again for continued bleeding. Continue until bleeding stops.

_____ **C-clamp Method:**

        _____ a. Apply pressure using the C-clamp.

        _____ b. Position the Plexiglas board under the patient to provide a firm surface to place the C-clamp on.

        _____ c. Position the C-clamp on the Plexiglas board but under the patient.

        _____ d. Attach the sterile disc to the tip of the compressor arm.

        _____ e. Position the C-clamp disc above the puncture site so that it can be lowered, with pressure applied, while the sheath is removed. Take care not to apply too much pressure before the sheath is out. This can cause a milking effect on any clot that is within the sheath.

        _____ f. Apply firm pressure above the puncture site until hemostasis is achieved. The RN will monitor the ECG for vasovagal responses.

        _____ g. Occlude dorsalis pedis pulse for 3 to 5 minutes. Then release just enough pressure to allow some blood flow to the foot. A slight pulse will be audible over the Doppler.

        _____ h. Release the pressure *slowly,* using the release level on the C-clamp, after 15 to 20 minutes. Watch for bleeding.

        _____ i. If bleeding continues, reapply the C-clamp.

        _____ j. Apply manual pressure if bleeding cannot be controlled with C-clamp.

_____ 15. Observe the site for 3 to 5 minutes before applying the butterfly dressing.

_____ 16. Document the patient's vital signs, pedal pulse checks, and dressing checks every 15 minutes for a half hour, then every 30 minutes for an hour, then every hour for 4 hours, and every 4 hours thereafter. Check under the dressing for bleeding.

_____ 17. Notify the RN immediately if you note any of the following: abnormalities in vital signs, chest pain, bleeding on dressing, hematoma, or diminished pedal pulses.

_____ 18. Instruct the patient to call for the RN for any of the following signs:

        _____ a. Signs of bleeding, feelings of warm blood oozing, or stickiness

        _____ b. Signs of compromised circulation—coolness, numbness, pain, dizziness

        _____ c. Signs of hematoma

        _____ d. Chest pain

_____ 19. Instruct the patient to remain flat in bed (or with the head of the bed up 15 degrees), usually for 4 to 6 hours. Then the patient can be up with assistance. The patient may be logrolled.

_____ 20. Remind the patient to apply firm pressure directly on the dressing over the insertion site whenever laughing, coughing, sneezing, bearing down, or tightening the abdominal muscles in any way.

_____ 21. Discard the dressings, sheath, and gloves in the appropriate medical waste container.

_____ 22. Document and report the results to the RN or preceptor.

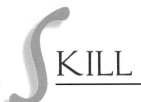

SKILL

Performing a Postcardiac Catheterization Check

Purpose A patient might require a cardiac catheterization for any of several reasons. A major purpose of cardiac catheterization is to determine the presence, location, and severity of any blockage to the arteries that supply blood to the heart. Catheterization is also performed to evaluate the function of the heart muscle and of the valves of the heart and to assess any damage to the heart from a heart attack, infection, or trauma. Finally, cardiac catheterization is often performed to assess the status of bypass surgery grafts.

The caregiver demonstrates the ability to do the following:

Objectives

1. Gather the correct supplies.

2. Communicate using a style that reduces the patient's anxiety.

3. Receive the patient after the catheterization.

4. Perform the postcardiac catheterization check.

5. Assist with patient care after the monitoring period is over.

6. Document observations appropriately.

7. Report the results of the procedure to the RN or preceptor.

Cardiac Catheterization A common technique for studying the structure and function of the heart. It allows the physician to view the blood supply to the heart and to view the various chambers and valves in the heart. Also called heart cath, coronary angiogram, arteriogram, and angiography.

Key Term

Gloves • Doppler machine • Doppler jelly • Washcloth

Supplies/
Equipment

- Cardiac catheterization is performed with a soft, narrow, flexible tube, or catheter.

Pertinent
Points

- The physician, usually a cardiologist, numbs the area that will be used. (The artery in the groin is usually selected, but the arm is another possible site.) The physician inserts the catheter into the artery and guides it into the heart. An X-ray dye is injected through the catheter into the heart so that the structures of the heart can be seen by X-ray. Patients often feel a warm, flushing feeling during this part of the procedure. When all of the X-ray pictures have been taken, the catheter is removed. Pressure is applied to the artery in the groin or arm for 10 to 20 minutes to allow the artery to close, and then a dressing is placed over the insertion site.

- Patients are not allowed to bend their leg or arm for a period of time after the test, and there will be specific activity restrictions.

- Patients are encouraged to drink fluids after the test to help flush the dye from their systems.

Age-Specific
Considerations

Due to the serious nature of this test, people of all ages are often nervous and anxious. Many of the patients who have this test are older adults. Keep the developmental factors of this age group in mind when providing care. Give step-by-step instructions when providing information. Speak in a low-pitched, clear voice. Be respectful. Provide for the patient's comfort and safety. While technological advances have come to be expected in the medical world, it is still a strange and often frightening environment for many patients.

> *T*he most important signs and symptoms to watch for during the post-cardiac catheterization check are discomfort, swelling, or bleeding at the catheter insertion site; chest pain; and numbness or coldness in the limb used for the test. The complications of cardiac catheterization are rare, but they must always be kept in mind. They include bleeding, allergic reaction, blood clot, infection, rhythm disturbance, injury to the heart, and death.

Steps

1. Wash hands.
2. Identify the patient and help move the patient from the stretcher to the bed.
3. Explain the procedure to the patient. Tell the patient what to expect during the postcardiac catheterization check (length of time for the check; frequency of vital signs; observation of the site and dressing, temperature, pallor of legs and feet; checking for pain, tingling in the leg, or chest pain; and the need to keep the leg or arm straight).
4. Obtain the patient's vital signs.
5. Obtain the dorsalis pedis and posterior tibial pulses.
6. Check the dressing for signs of bleeding or dried blood. Tell the patient to notify you or another caregiver immediately if bleeding occurs.
7. Check the insertion site for bleeding, bruising, swelling, and pain.
8. Check the extremity for color, mottling, and warmth. Ask the patient about any numbness or tingling.
9. Instruct the patient to remain on his or her back or supported by pillows toward the side where procedure was performed. The head of the bed may be elevated only to the degree indicated by the physician. Instruct the patient to apply pressure to the site when coughing or sneezing.
10. Help the RN position the patient to sit, stand, and then walk. This is the most common time for bleeding to occur. Patients should ambulate for 10 to 15 minutes before the pressure dressing and the IV are removed.
11. Document all observations on the flow sheet or patient record.
12. Report the following observations and complaints immediately to the nurse: a major change in blood pressure ($+/-$ 20 mmHg), bleeding at the insertion site, swelling at the site, tenderness or pain at the site, numbness or tingling in the leg or arm, chest pain, and the inability to urinate.

COMPETENCY VALIDATION

Skill: Performing a Postcardiac Catheterization Check

Name _____

Preceptor _____

Date _____

Competency Statement Performs a postcardiac catheterization check while demonstrating correct technique.

Not Competent: _____ 1. Is <u>unable to state reason</u> for task and <u>needs instructions</u> to perform task.

_____ 2. Understands reason for task but <u>needs instructions</u> to perform task.

Competent: _____ 3. Understands reason for task and is able to perform task but <u>needs to increase speed.</u>

_____ 4. Understands reason for task and is able to perform task <u>proficiently.</u>

Performance Criteria

The caregiver demonstrates the ability to do the following:

_____ 1. Wash hands.

_____ 2. Help move the patient from the stretcher to the bed.

_____ 3. Explain the procedure to the patient. Tell the patient what to expect during the postcardiac catheterization check (length of time for the check; frequency of vital signs; observation of the site and dressing, temperature, pallor of legs and feet; checking for pain, tingling in the leg, or chest pain; and the need to keep the leg or arm straight).

_____ 4. Obtain the patient's vital signs.

_____ 5. Obtain the dorsalis pedis and posterior tibial pulses.

_____ 6. Check the dressing for signs of bleeding or dried blood. Tell the patient to notify you or another caregiver immediately if bleeding occurs.

_____ 7. Check the insertion site for bleeding, bruising, swelling, and pain.

_____ 8. Check the extremity for color, mottling, and warmth. Ask the patient about any numbness or tingling.

_____ 9. Instruct the patient to remain on his or her back or affected side supported by pillows. The head of the bed may be elevated only to the degree indicated by the physician. Instruct the patient to apply pressure to the site when coughing or sneezing.

_____ 10. Help the RN position the patient to sit, stand, and then walk. This is the most common time for bleeding to occur. Patients should ambulate for 10 to 15 minutes before the pressure dressing and the IV are removed.

_____ 11. Document all observations on the flow sheet.

_____ 12. Report the following observations and complaints immediately to the nurse: a major change in blood pressure (+/− 20 mmHg), bleeding at the insertion site, swelling at the site, tenderness or pain at the site, numbness or tingling in the leg or arm, chest pain, and the inability to urinate.

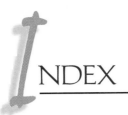

INDEX

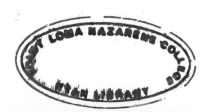